ONE PILL
Makes You Stronger

The Drug That Scorched My Soul

a memoir by
Jill Stegman

Transformation Media Books
Bloomington, Indiana

Copyright © 2019 Jill Stegman

All rights reserved. No part of this book may be reproduced or transmitted in any form or by any means, electronic or mechanical, including photocopying, recording, or by any information storage and retrieval system, without permission in writing from the publisher.

Published by Transformation Media Books, USA

www.TransformationMediaBooks.com
info@TransformationMediaBooks.com

An imprint of Pen & Publish, Inc.
www.PenandPublish.com
Bloomington, Indiana
(314) 827-6567

Print ISBN: 978-1-941799-62-8
eBook ISBN: 978-1-941799-63-5

Library of Congress Control Number: 2018953459

Printed on acid-free paper.

Author Note: I have recreated events, details, and conversations as accurately and truthfully as I can, based on my recollections. Names, locations, and identifying characteristics have been deliberately changed to protect the privacy of persons involved.

Contents

Preface: When I Knew	7
Chapter 1: Mr. Hyde	13
Chapter 2: An Unholy Union	23
Chapter 3: On Deaf Ears	35
Chapter 4: Respite	51
Chapter 5: November 11: The Devil Takes His Due	65
Chapter 6: The Facade	81
Chapter 7: Guilty as Charged	87
Chapter 8: Grief 101	93
Chapter 9: Time Online	103
Chapter 10: The Cure Is the Culprit	119
Chapter 11: The Battle	129
Chapter 12: Fault Lines	137
Chapter 13: Standard of Care	143
Chapter 14: The Road to Recovery	149
Chapter 15: Naked with Strangers	153
Chapter 16: Slowing Down the Race	157
Epilogue	165
Bibliography	167

"Love isn't there to make us happy. I believe it exists to show us how much we can endure."

—Hermann Hesse

Preface
When I Knew

My daughter Anna and I recently took in a matinée—a treat for both of us when she was home visiting. We had always gone to the neighborhood theater as a family. My husband was holder of the popcorn, while I sat on the other side of my kids, breaking up their whispering, which happened less often as they aged and started paying attention to the movie. Three years ago, I'd entered the same theater alone and waited for my husband to show up.

He never arrived.

* * *

It was a sun-soaked November day in 2013, normally a welcome prelude to a rainy California winter. But it only contrasted with my anxiety. I had waited for Don to come home all morning. We'd planned to see a matinée of *All Is Lost*, an adventure movie Don had chosen about a man who sails into a violent storm. For years Don was like the Robert Redford hero: weathered good looks, self-reliant, and superbly athletic. But he'd driven off in his truck hours ago, not saying where he was going. He'd never done that in all forty-three years of our marriage. I was used to at least a scribbled note, "Be back in a few hours," signed with a heart.

"I'm afraid of my feelings," he'd told me two days earlier, finally agreeing to seek help. This was coming from a man who'd charged up the street only one week after a knee replacement surgery.

I'd been calling psychiatrists when he drove off that morning. But I stopped calling after a few hours when all I got were messages: "The office will be closed from twelve o'clock until one o'clock. If this is an emergency, call nine-one-one." Was this an emergency? My husband had been gone all morning. Was that so unusual?

For us it was.

I went to the movie theater hoping Don would join me; he'd never stood me up before. "Only one ticket?" said the pleasant young woman behind the counter.

"Umm. . ." I looked around to see if Don had appeared. There were others waiting but the young ticket seller smiled without a sign of impatience.

Then it occurred to me that if Don came later, he might not have money. "Can I buy a ticket for my husband now and leave it with you?"

"Yes, I can do that for you. Tell him to ask for Miranda."

"That's a good idea," I said as if it was a brilliant suggestion. But I didn't know that his cell phone was lying on the table by our bed, announcing ten of my previous messages.

I took a seat in the back of the theater, where I could see Don when he arrived. Soon we'd be together like the other couples—murmuring, laughing, and sharing popcorn. How silly to think otherwise.

An older couple asked if the seat next to me was taken. "Yes, it is," I said. "My husband is just parking."

I wanted desperately to trade places with them—be living someone else's story. Why was I watching a movie when I was so worried about my husband? Wasn't he the one who worried about me? I never prayed, but I did that now, a generic "Help!" directed to any deity that might be listening. Anything to compete with the dread coiling tighter and tighter in my stomach.

I left my cell phone on; screw the message on the movie screen.

I scanned the lobby for Don one last time and missed the beginning of the movie. When I slipped into my seat, Robert Redford was somewhere in the Indian Ocean. A shipping crate had collided with his small yacht, and he was gluing pieces of fabric over a gaping hole. Redford reminded me of Don climbing our steeply sloped roof to repair a leak. How confidently he'd walked across the slippery tiles to find the source, a skylight.

The movie was a never-ending chain of calamities, and Redford calmly handled each one. His yacht was swamped and overturned by a wave, but he swam underneath, timing his movements just right to hop back on as the boat righted itself.

Don had once talked me into floating on inner tubes down the Merced River. Never one to pass up a new experience, Don looked longingly at the couples and families floating by while they drank beer and picnicked. "That looks like a blast. Let's try it."

I looked at the swiftly flowing water washing over and under fallen logs as the oblivious rafters swirled past. I sank to my default expression when embarking on one of my husband's "adventures."

"I don't know. What if I get stuck on one of those logs?"

But Don's enthusiasm won me over and he borrowed two inner tubes. "Steer clear of the middle, where the current is strongest." He pointed to a group of preteens spraying each other with squirt guns. "Like those guys."

But a rudder seemed to guide me straight into the middle of the river. I tried to get out of the current, but I was swept against a fallen tree and couldn't push myself away. I was trapped; the water sucking my legs under the log. "I can't hold on any longer," I screamed.

Don maneuvered swiftly over to me. Years of surfing and outdoor work on our property had strengthened his shoulder and back muscles. I was struck by his calmness and how quickly he calculated what had to be done.

He swam under the tree to break away any limbs that might have trapped me. "Just let the current pull you under," he shouted over the roar of the water. "You'll come up on the other side like I did." He said these words so calmly, like he was teaching me to ski.

I let go of my inner tube and when it popped up he grabbed it, and then I followed.

Now Redford had abandoned his sinking yacht, and he was adrift on a life raft. He learned how to use a sextant to chart his course to the shipping lanes. He discovered how to desalinate seawater. I understood why Don had chosen this movie about ingenuity in the face of disaster. My husband was a survivor, just like Redford. He'd even made it through cancer.

"Most would not have survived what you went through," said Don's doctor after the bone marrow transplant seven years ago, the graft-versus-host disease that followed, and the skin cancer that took his right ear.

After each incident, Don pressured the doctors immediately. "I just want to know how soon I can return to my normal activities." If the doctors said two weeks, Don would interpret it as five days. "I'll recover better if I'm not sitting around doing nothing," he said if I tried to stop him from grabbing his chain saw and scurrying up an oak tree.

I watched as Redford used all his flares but couldn't alert the giant cargo ships in his path, so he started a fire which engulfed his raft. He was forced to jump into the ocean. He floated under the water, holding his breath for what seemed an impossible amount of time. Then the screen went black. I thought the movie was over. But no, it couldn't be over. This was a Hollywood movie. The screen lit up. A faint light flickered above Redford, and a hand reached down through filtered light. Redford lifted his hand like Michelangelo's Adam reaching for the touch of God, for the spark of life. What did it matter that Adam represented youth and Redford was in his seventies? I was carried away by the outstretched hands reaching through the refracted rays—the scene fit my search for what was familiar, grasping at anything. I felt an inkling of hope, a slight relaxation of my twisting gut.

As the credits rolled, my cell phone buzzed—Don's name flashed as the caller.

"Hello," I shouted. I stumbled around knees and stomped on feet to get to the aisle, and then ran toward the exit.

"Mom?" It was Anna. I remembered that she was coming home from college for a visit.

I was nauseated by the double jolt of relief and disappointment. "Why are you calling on Dad's phone?"

"I lost mine." She sounded hurt at my tone. "I just wanted to let you know I got back from Santa Barbara."

"Is Dad there?"

"Why would I be calling you if Dad was here?" She sounded surly, but I was too overwhelmed to care.

"Shit. Fucking shit!" I screamed. What a fool I was to think I'd seen hope. The movie really ended with Redford floating just out of reach. He'd drowned, and the outstretched hand signified acceptance-of death. What else could *All Is Lost* mean?

I couldn't stop my own movie. All the clues I missed: the mysterious bag in the backseat holding an object shaped like a rifle. His mysterious disappearance just two days before and his excitement about where he'd been when he returned home. "I went to Whale Rock Reservoir," he'd said. "I'd forgotten how beautiful it is. You can see the ocean so clearly. I want to go back there with you tomorrow."

It was odd for Don to be so excited about a man-made lake surrounded by a sagging chain-link fence, and we'd driven by it many times, never stopping. But my relief that he wanted to do something with me overrode any misgivings. "Sure. I'd love to go there with you," I said.

"Momma?" Anna hadn't called me that since seventh grade. She'd never heard me swear.

Maternal instinct seeped through. I mustered a calm tone. "Honey, can you do something for me?" I said this in an overly sweet voice, the same one I used when she was eight and I wanted her to clean her room. "Dad's guns are under the front porch wrapped in a green blanket. Can you go check and tell me if you find them?"

"Why don't you look when you get home?" she said, wary of me now.

"It'll be dark then, and I just want to be sure they're still there." I didn't tell her I'd hidden them from Don.

She returned in a few minutes. "There's only one."

"Which one is it?"

"I don't know the difference. It's the one with the scope. What's going on? Where's Dad?"

She had found the twenty-two, which meant Don had the shotgun.

Chapter 1
Mr. Hyde

Six months earlier I had a husband who went bike riding with me on the rim of the Grand Canyon at sunrise. We kayaked down the coast of Kauai into Hanalei Bay. We shared a love of pad Thai and Japanese architecture.

We visited the Huntington Library in Los Angeles in 1970 and admired the openness and transparency of the traditional Japanese home located on the grounds—its simple lines and gardens in sync with nature.

"I want to live in a house like this," I said, pushing back one of the sliding screens.

Don pulled me close. "I want to make love in this house."

I laughed. "It's not very private in here. The rooms are all interconnected."

"We'll have to modify it a little," Don murmured into my hair. "Make our bedroom more private." He slid his hand under my peasant top.

"Our house? Our bedroom? That sounds like a long-term plan." I looked into his deep-set eyes that always fascinated me—they changed colors with his mood. Now they were a mesmerizing blue-green shade.

Don held me at arm's length with a look of mock concern. "Wait a minute. Are you proposing to me?"

"No way. I said I liked the house and you started talking about us living in a house like this."

Don pulled me to him again. "In that case, if we're going to be living in the same house and we love each other, then maybe we should get married."

I put my arms around his neck. "So, is this a proposal?"

"Yep," he said nuzzling my ear. "But you're the one who brought it up talking about privacy."

We eventually built our own home in Atascadero in 1987, on the central coast of California, based on the Japanese style, using glass and filtered light, a world which opens wide to nature. The view from our deck looked over an oak-filled valley backed by a ridge where coastal fog ambled over and poured down the slopes like a waterfall. Sunsets stretched, long and luminously grazing the ridge top, reminding us of all the years we had together.

Everything was according to plan. We'd moved from the crowds and congestion of Santa Monica to San Diego. And when San Diego's housing developments began spreading ominously through the open spaces we loved, we moved to Atascadero, a small rural town. Don taught social studies at a middle school nearby, and I was a librarian at the local high school.

We raised our children, John and Anna, with our love of the natural world and its inhabitants. Local hikes, or "forced marches," as our children referred to them, were a part of family life. John and Anna both incorporated a love of nature into their lives. They would rather be outside looking at stars than watching TV. John wanted to become an environmental lawyer.

Don was our protector and instigator of adventure. When we went snorkeling in Hawaii, he always found the best places to swim with dolphins, which meant walking a mile or so to an isolated cove far away from other families. We hiked through a rain forest for three miles to get to the best vantage point to view a volcanic eruption.

What I loved most about Don was his devotion. During our first years of marriage, I came home dazed and exhausted from my forty-five-minute drive in LA traffic commuting to my data-entry job, wanting to crawl into bed and take a nap before dinner.

"You're not physically tired, you're mentally and emotionally drained and exercise will help you feel better, get those endorphins going," he would say, rolling bikes out of the garage.

At first I looked at the bike skeptically. I hadn't ridden one since I was ten. "How is exercise going to make me feel less tired?"

He handed me a pair of bike shorts and an outrageous fluorescent-pink shirt. "Just give it a try. We'll start out with thirty minutes a day. If you don't like it, I'll take this stuff back."

He was right. The exuberance and thrill of bike riding was a life-changing experience, and Don was delighted when I began riding every day after work. It led to the purchase of several more bikes and many more outdoor sports we did together.

One-time, cross-country skiing in Sequoia National Park, we got caught in a whiteout from a freak blizzard. I couldn't see anything at all, not even my hand when I held it directly in front of my face. I was scared and mad at Don for talking me into coming here; there was supposedly an easier route off the main trail. He had been right behind me, but I had no idea how far away he was.

I felt him tug on my arm. Then he guided me to a log. I was shaking. "How are we going to get out of here? I can't see anything."

He held my hand. "Don't be scared." His voice sounded close, but I couldn't see him. "It's just a whiteout. This happens sometimes when you get into some clouds at this elevation. The clouds block out the sun and blend into the snow. This is just a bit of a snow flurry, not a real blizzard. It'll pass in a few minutes." And, of course, it did.

The milestones came and went: Don drove to Central Juvenile Hall in downtown LA employed as a probation officer, and then went back to graduate school to become a school psychologist while I worked as a marketing research assistant. We moved from Santa Monica because the Los Angeles area was not conducive to the outdoor activities we enjoyed. In San Diego, Don worked as a school psychologist while I went to graduate school to become a teacher.

After we'd been living in San Diego for five years, Don decided he wanted to teach. "I can work better with these kids and their learning and behavior problems as their teacher." He obtained his credentials and taught children with learning disabilities, and then switched to social studies in a regular classroom when we moved to Atascadero.

Jobs, houses, children: we had everything we wanted. In between were ferocious conflicts, of course, two different notions of the right route to take. After driving secondhand and even fourth-hand vehicles all my life, I decided that I wanted a new car when I turned fifty. Don didn't agree.

"It's just a waste of money, and they're too expensive. We can't afford it." When he decided something, his face seemed chiseled from stone, like the figures on Mount Rushmore.

"We can make payments like most people. We don't have to pay in cash."

"I don't want to pay interest. You can buy two or three used cars for what a new one costs."

"I know, but used cars break down all the time. We've been married for thirty years, and we've had fifteen used cars that have all been driven into the ground. God knows what they've cost us in repairs. I'm tired of breaking down and getting towed. It's not safe for me or the kids."

Mentioning safety seemed to soften him. We went back and forth like this for a month until one day he said, "All right, get your new car! But at least get something that won't fall apart at seventy-five thousand miles."

I bought a Volkswagen Passat, still running with two hundred fifty thousand miles. "That was one of the best things we ever did," Don said after we'd had the car for ten years. We were at a restaurant celebrating our anniversary. He raised his champagne glass. "Here's to you, Sweets."

We'd made it to our fortieth wedding anniversary, and when we imagined the end of our lives, we saw each other in the same bed.

The milestones faded into vague memories in 2007 when Don had a bone marrow transplant for a blood cancer disease. We were living in an apartment across the street from Maynard Hospital because Don had to be monitored for three months during his recovery. He had just been released from the hospital, after being isolated in his room for a month to prevent infections due to his depleted immune system. It had been a terrible trial for Don. He was allowed outside his room wearing a respirator. He couldn't go outdoors at all because he was vulnerable to infections. The sun, which had been his joy and comfort, became toxic.

I came by every day to walk with him up and down the hospital hallways. Don, wearing his "Darth Vader" mask, pushed the rig that held his oxygen tubes. He waved at nurses and hospital staff and introduced me as his girlfriend. He told everyone, "I want to be the poster child of the bone marrow transplant unit." He bargained for a stationary bike in his room so that he could exercise without the respirator.

When it was time for me to leave the hospital and return to our apartment, his attitude changed. Sometimes he'd shove furniture around or punch a wall. "I have to get my ass out of here."

"The doctors are saying you're doing really well, so it should be soon."

"They said a month and that's how long I've been here."

"No, they said at least a month after your chemo treatments."

"I'll ask Dr. Lin tomorrow."

Dr. Lin was Don's oncologist. She'd advocated for Don's bone marrow transplant when it was generally not performed on people over fifty-five. Small and crisp in her tailored clothing, she projected confidence and warmth. Highly respected, Dr. Lin, MD and PhD, walked around the hospital followed by an entourage of medical students and visiting doctors. She had supervised bone marrow transplants for over twenty-five years.

Don was released the next week to our apartment near the hospital with fifteen different prescriptions. He immediately prepared to walk outside wearing the respirator mask, which would be required for several more weeks. His muscular legs had not atrophied much from the long hospital stay, and he looked athletic and fit striding down the street. I imagined him back on the tennis courts within two weeks.

He returned in only a half hour, limping, grimacing with every step. He winced when he pulled off his bloody socks. Three-inch wide blisters covered his feet and ankles. We drove in silence to the clinic, the car filled with oppressive anxiety. Don had recovered well in the hospital, and it was disappointing for him to return so quickly.

We knew the risk for complications was highest during the first hundred days post-transplant, especially for the dreaded graft-versus-host disease (GVHD), when the patient's immune system fights with the donor's introduced blood.

Dr. Lin walked into the clinic flanked by her retinue of medical students. They crowded around while Dr. Lin lifted each of Don's tortured feet to examine the sores. "This looks like graft-versus-host disease of the skin." The other doctors leaned in for a closer look. "Mr. Stegman is thirty-one days post-transplant, which puts him in the critical time period for developing GVHD."

She looked at Don and spoke to him calmly and directly. Dr. Lin was thorough, leaving nothing assumed. "GVHD happens when the white blood cells from your donor and your own immune system fight each other. Your resistance is lowered right now through the chemo treatments, but it's still strong enough to do battle with the donor. The graft is the donor and you are the host," she continued as Don lay back with his eyes closed, in obvious pain. "The white blood cells are like drone bees protecting their queen. They'll fight to the death. We have to calm them down until they accept each other. That's what prednisone does. It's the main drug we have that can fight GVHD."

Dr. Lin explained the physical side effects of the steroid prednisone—diabetes, bloating, and high blood pressure.

"Patients have been known to have some emotional issues as well," she added.

Don was prescribed 160 milligrams a day of the drug, the highest recommended dosage. Little did we know that his deal with the devil had begun. In fact, I would face down this devil each day for the next seven years.

By "emotional issues," I expected sadness, maybe some irritability. Instead, the changes turned his behavior upside down. He stopped going outside because he was afraid of getting an infection. He declared that the maintenance worker, who cleaned the pool and cared for the shrubbery around the apartment complex, was really a thief. "I think he's trying to case the place," Don said, standing by the window. "You never see him doing anything but watching people."

As a trained counselor and psychologist, the real Don would have rolled his eyes at this bizarre behavior. But the real Don had vanished.

One night I woke up to find Don gone, and I discovered him outside in his pajamas turning door handles on the other apartments on our floor.

"What are you doing out here in the middle of the night?" I wondered if sleep-walking was another side effect of prednisone.

He looked at me with a puzzled expression. "I'm trying to get some clean sheets, but these doors are all locked. The nurses never lock these doors." After that I slept on a mattress by the front door.

The doctors and nurses at the clinic laughed at my stories about Don's irrational behavior. "Everyone is a bit loopy on prednisone," was the stock answer.

But this wasn't just loopy. The hallucinations turned to paranoia, and Don refused to shower because he was afraid it would make his skin condition worse. The GVHD had affected the rest of his body. For weeks, he wore the same T-shirt, glued to his back from the weeping blisters. He would only leave the apartment for clinic appointments, and he didn't want me to leave either. I continued to go along with his weirdness because the medical staff acted like his behavior was normal.

One day we had an argument about me leaving the apartment to go for a walk. Don blocked the door. "No, I don't want you to go outside where I can't see you."

Since Don had deteriorated so much physically and mentally, I'd stopped exercising as well, not wanting to leave him alone for very long. I wasn't taking care of myself. I'd gained weight and I needed physical activity. The complex's swimming pool was directly below our third-story window. "How about if I swim and you can watch me from up here?"

"How long will you be gone?" Don said, his eyes darting nervously from me to the window.

"How about a half hour? You can time me and wave. I'll come back."

I saw him at the window watching me stroke back and forth in the pool, and this is how I got my exercise every day for a month. We had a routine: after I left, Don would immediately set the timer and lock the door behind me. When the timer went off, Don waved and yelled if I didn't instantly get out of the pool. Don gave me five minutes to return. He'd quickly lock the door again after I was inside.

Our world shrank to the tiny capsule of our apartment, and our social life consisted of daily visits to the clinic. The nurses and doctors seemed very competent, and I trusted them even though I was growing increasingly alarmed about Don's physical and mental state.

Dr. Johnson oversaw him at the clinic while Dr. Lin rotated to the hospital. She didn't have Dr. Lin's warmth. When she saw Don in the clinic, she examined him like a lab specimen, taking photos of his peeling wounds for her research report. I had to look up what she said on the internet. "Maculopapular rash and generalized erythroderma with bilious formation, often with desquamation," meant that Don's skin was blistering and sloughing off over 90 percent of his body.

I started leaving Don at the clinic so that I had an hour alone. Shopping was easier without him; he tended to wander off at the market. One time I found him by the freezer, opening cartons of ice cream bars. "I'm looking for those raspberry ones I like," he said.

I occasionally took walks through the pristine residential neighborhoods of million-dollar homes. Leaves from the deciduous trees floated down and covered the lawns and sidewalks, and I could crunch through them if I was lucky enough to get to them before the gardeners and street cleaners. I'd never been in a neighborhood of California so reminiscent of fall color, and I wanted to walk on and on to savor the new experience.

One time I got lost and was late getting back to the clinic. Don was waiting for me outside the sliding doors holding a cane. He looked like an alien wearing his respirator. He wore slip-on canvas shoes with the toes cut out to accommodate his blistered feet. I realized what a chore it was for him to walk even across the street to the clinic. It was heartbreaking to see him this way.

Don refused to get out of bed one morning. "Just get me to the hospital," he said. "Dr. Lin will take care of me."

The hospital doors opened with a pneumatic hiss and Don shuffled to the BMT unit, clinging to my arm, and collapsed, sobbing. Dr. Lin was obviously shocked by Don's appearance. She hadn't seen him since he was first discharged from the hospital—when we had left in such high spirits. His peeling eyelids and bulging eyeballs made him look particularly ghoulish. She looked down at him slumped against the wall. "Mr. Stegman, what's wrong?"

Don stared ahead and wailed. "All I know is that my name is Don."

The intake report from that day noted that Don was admitted for "prednisone psychosis," and grade 4 GVHD. How severe was grade 4 GVHD? I hurried home to Google it and discovered grade 4 was the most severe form and was considered life-threatening. If the disease wasn't stopped soon, his other vital organs would be attacked. His liver and kidneys would fail. He would die.

Dr. Lin brought Don back from death's doorstep with some very specialized treatments for his GVHD, which included photopheresis, a transfusion-type of procedure involving an intravenous

Mr. Hyde

injection. The drugs Haldol and Ativan were prescribed for the psychosis. Don would be treated with prednisone many times over the next seven years for the GVHD flare-ups, but this was the only time Dr. Lin treated him for the mental issues related to steroids.

During these periods I braced myself for a change in his personality, the usual irritability and impatience, but he never became psychotic again. As Don survived each episode of the GVHD, including an attack on his liver, he rebounded quickly and soon the GVHD was under control. He was still visiting the hospital every two months for his photopheresis treatment, always asking Dr. Lin when he would be off all the medications.

"I feel like a dog on a chain," he said during one of his appointments. "How long will I be on drugs? It's been four years now."

Dr. Lin examined Don's mouth, looking for tell-tale signs of GVHD: sore spots on the tongue and throat. "It looks good now, but it depends on how you do in the next year. GVHD usually burns itself out after five years."

"So, in five years I won't be on any drugs?"

"Well, you'll probably always be on a low dose of prednisone as a preventative measure because you've had so many episodes of GVHD."

"Can I quote you on that?" Don said. His eyes looked serious, despite his smile.

But six years after his bone marrow transplant, when we thought we should be done with GVHD, Don developed GVHD pneumonia and was prescribed 90 milligrams of prednisone a day.

This time my loving and devoted husband of forty-two years became a monstrous, horror-movie villain. It was as if someone was tinkering with his brain, manipulating him to say and do the vilest things completely antithetical to his normal, good-natured personality. Don's voice changed, his speech became pressured and distorted. I knew it was the prednisone, but I didn't know what to do. He slammed his fists on the table when I suggested that he ask his doctors what was wrong. "It's you who has the problem."

One night we sat down to one of Don's favorite dinners of chicken cacciatore, mashed potatoes, and salad. He took a few bites and then put his fork down.

"This tastes funny. What did you put into this?"

Usually Don was complimentary about my cooking, so I wondered if this was a new side effect of prednisone. "It's the same way I've always cooked this dish. I didn't do anything differently."

Don acted offended, like I'd purposely served him something inedible. "I can't eat this. It has a chemical taste." He picked up his plate and threw the food in the trash. He went out and came back with a chicken wrap from McDonald's.

After a week of this same behavior at meals, I stopped cooking for us. Don began buying take-out meals and eating by himself outside on the deck, away from me. At first, I tried to coax him back in.

"Come on back inside and talk to me. Tell me what I've done."

"No, I can't talk to you without arguing. It upsets my stomach. Just leave me the alone."

"What is wrong with Dad?" I asked Anna, who was home from college. "He's never been this bad on prednisone before."

"I don't know what's wrong," said Anna, "but that man out there isn't Dad."

We'd always sat down to dinner as a family. John and Anna, now in their twenties, still recited in unison how, no matter what, "You were expected to be home at dinnertime unless you gave twenty-four-hour notice." These had been the cherished times where our family weighed in on the events of the day. Don's callous disregard of this special tradition made me feel isolated and deeply anxious about our marriage, my foundation. And his disdain for me was astounding; he seemed irritated by my very presence.

Our years of family dinners representing a steadfast companionship were just hazy memories. What I'd taken for granted, a life with my soul mate of forty-two years, was being dismantled with ferocious speed. Every morning brought a new incident to reinforce my anxiety.

Chapter 2
An Unholy Union

But the disappearance of the family meal time was nothing compared to our ill-fated house-hunting trip. Don had heard from a friend about how inexpensive houses were in Ohio and decided we needed some investments to make our pensions go further. He wanted to take our savings and buy rental houses.

But he knew nothing about investing in real estate. Mania, I later learned, was a side effect of prednisone. The euphoria imbued him with great confidence. In this state, he thought he could accomplish anything. He read how-to books and followed real estate blogs full of questionable advice about buying foreclosures. He became an insomniac, staying up nights "becoming an expert" on the real estate market.

He never appeared to question that he was becoming another person. He had never been interested in real estate investing or any investments. I kept hoping that he would burn out on this folly and turn to a new interest to absorb his insatiable energy.

When Don began talking about the rust-belt town of Youngstown, located on the Ohio–Pennsylvania border, I knew this was not a passing phase. He'd even found a real estate agent who claimed there were "good deals" to be found for ten thousand dollars. I worried about him going off on this far-flung trip. He'd always been so conservative about our finances, leaving me to handle most of the investments, but I didn't trust him now.

I decided to go with him after I Googled Youngstown and discovered that it had succumbed to the ravages of post-industrialization—its whole economy had been built on the steel industry, and when steel pulled out, fifty thousand workers lost their jobs. The town now had one of the highest poverty rates in the nation. The huge 1930s houses Don had discovered online were being offered for only a few thousand dollars, but there were no buyers. Some *were* actually being given away.

I showed the list to Don. "I don't feel good about this place," I said. "It sounds like no one wants to live there, so how are we going to get any renters?'

"Bullshit on the bastards who wrote this." Don balled up the printout and threw it in the trash. "They probably made it sound bad because they don't want outside investors coming in. My real estate agent assured me there were good neighborhoods in Youngstown. You can stay home if you want, but I'm going to Ohio."

The idea of Don loose in Ohio buying houses with our retirement savings overrode my fears. By now, we seemed thrown together in an unholy union, a match of opposites. The slightest hesitation on my part to anything Don suggested brought a harsh reaction. He'd slammed our bedroom door so often it had cracked at the hinges. I had no choice but to go with him.

Prednisone was a devil I needed to confront head on.

By the time we arrived in Ohio, Don had a list of houses for sale. While we waited for the real estate agent at the first house, Don devised his own method of house hunting. He said, "Canvassing was the best way to get to know the neighborhood." His "uniform" for the occasion was an old Hawaiian shirt and jeans. The years since his bone marrow transplant had taken a toll on his appearance. His once-thick hair had grown back thin and sparse from the chemotherapy and he had scars from a virulent cancer that had taken his right ear. The high dose of prednisone also caused bloating. A moon face had softened the angular jawline. He used to be very concerned about his appearance, and he also looked very neat whether dressed for tennis or the farmer's market. He never wanted to be thought of as tacky.

"Maybe you should dress more like a professional," I said. "You could wear that blue button-down shirt you used to wear to school. And you have those nice Dockers."

"I don't want to look too dressed up," he said. "People in areas like this don't trust you if you look better than they do. I want to meet them at their level."

Don walked the street, talking to random people who happened to be out and about. I held back. At first it was amusing to observe Don. He walked right up and introduced himself, and he was usually well received. People stopped mowing their lawns or hauling in groceries to chat. An elderly couple sitting on their porch not only told Don about the neighborhood, but everything they knew about the house for sale and its past and present occupants. "The Hudsons had the fence put up after they were robbed ten years ago." They offered Don coffee, and he gestured for me to come over. I shook my head vigorously from my vantage point beside the car, making as if we had to go.

A young man came down the sidewalk toward me with a pit bull on a leash. When he passed I saw that his arms and neck were covered with tattoos—crudely drawn knives dripping blood, intermingled with skulls and crossbones. Don intercepted him for an interview. "I'm thinking of buying a house here. What do you think of this neighborhood?"

The man looked around uneasily.

Don was determined to get a response. "That's a beautiful dog. Can I pet him?"

When Don leaned down to touch the dog the man stepped back. "Don't come any closer or he'll rip your throat out, and I ain't shittin' you." The dog sprang forward in combat mode, and Don raised his hands and backed away.

"He was probably just a drug dealer, not someone from around here," Don said as the man and dog continued down the sidewalk past a vacant house with bashed-out windows.

A police car was parked across the street; an officer sat inside, casually drinking coffee. Don strolled over, and I trailed behind rather than standing alone. We had drawn attention from the neighbors.

Don introduced himself. "So, what's this area like in terms of crime? Would you say it's safe?"

The officer put down his coffee cup and regarded Don warily. "This is a shitty area in a shitty town," he said, before a call came through and he sped away.

"Maybe Ohio isn't a good place for us to invest?" Youngstown felt like a foreign country, and I was way out of my comfort zone. I wanted to go home.

But Don seemed unfazed. "We have to at least wait for the real estate agent and take a look inside some of these places. I came here to buy some goddamned houses."

Don headed to a bar and pizza joint on the corner where he planned to "interview" the owner. I trailed my requisite few feet behind. A few angry-looking young men slouched against the building, smoking various substances and squinting in the sun. The pit bull from the encounter before was tied to a bicycle rack guarding its three-foot circumference of the sidewalk. Don greeted the men outside with a friendly nod. He had a six-inch scar from a cancer operation that ran from his right ear to his jugular, and the men could have mistaken him for a street fighter, or they could have recognized Don's steroid-infused glare. Surprisingly, they nodded back respectfully.

I had a choice: accompany Don into the darkness, where more drinking than eating was going on, or wait outside with the scowling young men and the pit bull. I decided to use the bathroom. When I came out, Don was waiting for me, holding a slab of pizza. "The owner said it was a pretty nice area. I'm going back to meet the agent."

When the real estate agent failed to appear, I hoped that was the end of it. But Don decided to contact the residents himself and walked up to the first house. Since the for sale sign read "Do Not Disturb the Occupants," I didn't think we'd be very well received, and I didn't want to encounter another pit bull or ill will. But Don was already knocking and ringing the bell. "I'm not going to let a real estate agent who can't even do his job stand in my way."

A middle-aged couple answered the door and Don instantly became Mr. Charm. He introduced himself to Ella Mae and Jim as someone "looking to move to Ohio," and told them he was considering buying the house and what did they think of the place? "I want to know everything." Since they were renters they eagerly let him in to show all the problems with the house from minor holes in the wall to severe basement leaks. Don assured them that he would "take care of everything" and that he wasn't going to be a "slum lord."

Later, when I questioned the logic of making promises when we didn't know what the repairs would cost or if we were even buying the property, Don became angry. "What's your problem? You're always holding me back. I should have just come by myself."

We clashed for the rest of the day while driving through one depressed neighborhood after another. I wanted to go back home, and Don insisted on staying until we found a house. Our situation devolved into a pathetic scenario when I demanded to be taken to the airport, and Don refused.

"Stop!" I screamed as he picked up speed, going fifty-five in a twenty-five zone. The houses and street corners became a gray blur. "Let me drive!"

"No," he said, clamping his fingers more tightly on the wheel.

"Then let me out." I grabbed the armrest. "You're trying to kill us."

Don slammed on the brakes and I fell forward. The seatbelt dug across my neck. He looked at me with a malevolent sneer. "So get the fuck out if you want."

I jumped out of the car, tottering to the curb on my platform sandals in the middle of what had been downtown Youngstown. I tucked in my blouse and started walking toward a small market with sham confidence. I'd made my ridiculous demand and there was no going back. I would find my own way to California.

I trudged along the streets looking for a bus stop. There were none. The city center seemed to be abandoned. It was trashed out, eerie and forbidding, sirens in the distance and a few of the ubiquitous pizza/bar establishments scattered among blocks of vacant stores and businesses. People pushed shopping carts filled with clothing and sleeping bags or rifled through trash cans. If anything, I wanted to be invisible. The idea of getting out of Youngstown by myself was way too complicated and dangerous for me to fathom. I never imagined, after over forty years of marriage, that I'd be abandoned in such a place.

Don had been tailing me in the car, ignoring my glares and angry gestures to move on. He wasn't mad enough or crazy enough to abandon me just yet. His protective instincts were still intact, a sliver of light penetrating the prednisone fog. He found me in a phone booth, which held nothing but a soggy directory plastered to the floor and a few dangling wires. My last idea had been to call information and ask for the number to the bus station or cab service. My cell phone battery had died. Don leaned over and opened the passenger door. I slumped in and we drove off without speaking. It was as if we both realized that the silence was a prelude for what was to come. In our doomed relationship, we would retreat into our own worlds.

* * *

It was getting late in Youngstown, and we spent an hour driving past boarded-up motels and glazed-eyed people who seemed to have no apparent ambition but waiting for something to happen. I was eventually able to find a motel online on Don's phone and made a reservation. It was near a police station, which I hoped meant it was safe.

Don had become increasingly agitated as we saw one run-down place after another. We were both stunned by what we'd seen—mostly elderly and disabled people living in 1920s-era, two-story houses with no stair railings, broken windows, leaking pipes, and fifty-year-old furnaces.

Just when I thought parts of the old Don were breaking through the prednisone, Don came out swinging. The clerk told us we were charged an extra fee for making the reservation on the internet.

"We weren't told this at the time," Don shouted at the young woman. "This is bullshit."

Seeing where this interaction was going, I tried to defuse Don's anger. "It's my fault. I probably didn't read the terms and conditions." Anything to avert the disaster I saw brewing.

But this made Don angrier. "We shouldn't have to pay just because we made reservations on the internet. We want our money back."

The clerk looked like she'd rather be anywhere but here dealing with this enraged man, but she told Don she couldn't give him a refund. "But I can have my manager call you."

"It's not that much extra," I said.

Don exploded. "I'm not staying at this fucking dump with their cheap-shit rules." He grabbed his bag and slammed through the doors. I saw him outside yelling and gesturing at a woman standing on the lawn smoking a cigarette, and then he got in the car and drove away. I began a mumbled apology to the hotel clerk when the woman from outside burst through the doors and stormed up to me.

"I'm calling the cops on that asshole. Is he on meth? I was just standing there having a smoke and he gave me a look, called me a lazy-ass bitch."

No excuse about how "my husband is on medication," was going to lessen the anger and hostility. I couldn't offer a defense for Don's appalling behavior anymore. There was no denying that something was terribly wrong with him, and I wasn't capable of fixing this situation. I gave in and let the tears stream down my face. "I'm sorry my husband is acting this way. I don't know what's wrong with him. If you really feel that you need to call the police, then go ahead."

The two women looked at me with pity, like I was a victim. This, they understood. I didn't see myself as an abused wife. Don had never struck me, although I certainly felt battered. I couldn't pretend any longer that I was coping. The clerk produced a box of tissues from behind the counter.

The other woman took a handful of the tissues and gave them to me. "Well, I'm not going to call the cops," she said as I dabbed my eyes. "But it's only because of you, not that bastard. Once you get settled in, why don't you come down to the bar and we'll talk. I'm working until two."

I was grateful and touched by her offer, but I didn't want sympathy or to cry on a stranger's shoulder in some bar. What I really wanted was to retreat to a dark place and to have someone rescue me the way Don used to.

I sat in my hotel room trying to make sense of the events of the day. I had no reference for what was happening, and no one to go to for help. My life with Don had become frightening, and my method of dealing with him was completely ineffective. I couldn't take him on at this level.

I called Don and he answered. He'd gotten a room at a motel nearby and was waiting for my call, for me to make the first move. I had to be the one to give in, and I had to play the game his way. I said I wanted to go home. He wanted to stay and keep looking for houses. I agreed because at least I would have a reprieve from him for a few extra weeks. He still had symptoms of pneumonia—shortness of breath and fatigue—and had postponed his scheduled appointment with Dr. Lin and Dr. Major to remain in Ohio.

Dr. Lin knew Don's history with prednisone and Dr. Major must have had access to his medical records. He was supposed to see them both when he returned. They would understand how bad he was and know what to do, and our life would return to normal.

Don called a week after I got home to Atascadero. In the brief hiatus away from him, I'd created a fantasy world, made myself almost believe I was single, following an unscripted pattern of activities. But when I heard his voice on the phone and his weird, pressured speech, I remembered that my life hadn't changed. I was back in this nightmare.

    I couldn't make out much of the conversation because he kept interrupting my questions. From what I understood, he had given up on Youngstown after he talked to a man who was bulldozing an entire block of 1930s-era houses like the ones we had seen. Don talked about conducting an on-the-spot "interview" with the man, who got down from his bulldozer to give a crash course on the Ohio real estate market: "We're taking down these houses because no one wants to live here anymore because there's no work. The houses stay vacant and the rats and druggies move in. My advice on buying rentals is to stay away from the big cities and go to the suburbs."

    Somehow Don wound up in Piqua, a suburb of Dayton, five hours from Youngstown, after he'd gotten a "lead" from someone he met in McDonald's. Foreclosures were the norm, though Piqua was no Youngstown. It was down, but not out, only waiting for a breath of fresh air. Don got a reference for a real estate agent named Sue Wray from the owner of an ice-cream shop in Piqua. Sue was a cancer survivor with a big heart and great patience. She must have noticed that Don was off-kilter, must have witnessed a few rages and irrational acts. But something in her personality calmed Don. She was able to work with him and accomplish what I couldn't—managing his mania and mood disorder to a positive end. She referred to Don later as "the most focused person I ever met. He was always nice to me. I never would have thought he had a mental illness."

    With her real estate acumen and Don's relentless obsession, they found two properties for ten and twenty thousand dollars. I hoped that the purchase of the houses would calm down the mania and accompanying agitation. I was jealous of the way Don waxed so enthusiastically about Sue Wray and what she'd done for him while I'd failed. Don hadn't just been lucky, his instincts about "interviewing," heightened self-confidence, and ferocious motivation had ultimately benefited us, all driven by the prednisone. But at what cost?

Don came home from Ohio victorious, but the experience had taken a toll on his health. For months he'd only been sleeping a few hours a night. He struggled with his backpack when I picked him up at the airport and asked me to carry it, acting like I should have offered: "Can you give me a little help here?" Prednisone had taken a toll on him physically as well—he'd lost muscle mass. The slack skin on his upper arms, which had once covered lean and muscular biceps, stretched over brittle bones, and his well-developed pectoral muscles had flattened. When I greeted him, it felt like I was hugging a skeleton.

We headed up to Maynard the next day, a three-hour drive north, for the long-postponed appointments with Dr. Lin and Dr. Major, the pulmonary specialist.

In the waiting room, a man was talking loudly on his cell phone. After the conversation continued for several minutes, Don jumped up from his chair.

"Do you mind taking that call outside?"

I hoped that this would end it. Don had come across politely and any reasonable person would have agreed to his request.

The man took the phone from his ear. He was tall and obese with a protruding belly. He looked like a football player gone to seed. "Why should I? I have a right to make calls. I'm waiting for my doctor to call me in and I need to take this." He turned away from Don and continued talking on his phone.

"Can you at least lower your voice? Everyone in this entire room can hear you."

"Who are you to tell me what I can and can't do? I don't see any rules here about not talking on phones."

Intervening would only make matters worse. I got up and went to the receptionist, who was ensconced behind a glass partition. "How much longer does Don Stegman have to wait?"

I must have looked panicked because the receptionist said, "Just a minute," and left to check with the nursing assistant. She quickly returned, "We can take him next." She looked past me. The argument between Don and the man on the phone was escalating.

By now, Don was red-faced and snarling. "Put that goddamn phone away." The man flipped Don off and continued his phone conversation. I kept hoping that Don would be called in before a security guard appeared. Then, again a security guard might take notes on the incident, which might influence the doctors to intervene.

The other patients had stopped reading their newspapers and books to observe the drama. Don looked back at them with a what-are-we-going-to-do-now? expression. He took out his phone and started playing sixties rock music. He held his device next to the guy's ear and let the Rolling Stone's "Jumpin' Jack Flash" blast loudly enough to drown out any conversation. The man tried to push Don's arm away, but Don was too fast for him. He easily dodged the furious attempts by switching his phone from one hand to the other as the guy tried to slap it away. But he was too heavy to keep up with Don's antics. He was soon sweating heavily and out of breath.

"Mr. Donald Stegman?"

An older nursing assistant with a military bearing, wearing glasses on a chain around her neck, was calling for Don's appointment. The woman possessed some magical power that broke the tension. Don dropped his arm and followed dutifully behind as she led us down the hallway.

Dr. Major was waiting for us in the examination room. He was a brilliant young doctor who was adept at diagnosing lung diseases from the vague scattering of dark pinpoints and shadowy areas on X-rays. He was not impressed with Don's house-hunting spree. "This expedition has taken a toll on your health."

Dr. Major flicked on the TV screen and shook his head when he saw the labs and chest X-rays. A milky cloud covered nearly 50 percent of Don's lungs. He was very ill with cryptogenic organizing pneumonia, and more prednisone was prescribed. I'd hoped that the doctor would have been prompted to question Don's mental health after the incident in the waiting room, which he must have known about, but nothing was prescribed except Ambien to help with sleeping. No note was made of Don's pressured speech and extreme irritability.

Dr. Lin came in next with a scolding expression. "Mr. Stegman, you have not been following the doctor's orders. You have to rest now and not push yourself so that you can recover."

Much to my disappointment Don didn't yell back at her or show any sign of anger. He looked abashed and said nothing. I had to say something. "He's having problems controlling his anger. I tried to get him to come home. Something is really wrong with Don. Isn't there something . . . ?"

All three stared at me, the doctors folded their arms. Don's look was menacing. There was an awkward silence.

Dr. Lin walked to the door. "I think we should just worry about getting Mr. Stegman's physical health back right now, and then we can consider tapering him off the prednisone."

Dr. Major nodded. I didn't expect him to disagree.

Chapter 3
On Deaf Ears

The increase in prednisone helped Don's pneumonia but made his mania and mood even worse. In 2013, seven years after his bone marrow transplant, he had been on high doses of 90 milligrams for the past four months. Our bikes sat in the garage collecting cobwebs. Don didn't have the strength to ride, nor did he want to ride with me. He looked haggard and beat down. One time I came back from a walk to find Don up an oak tree cutting limbs with a chain saw. He'd climbed a rickety ladder to get there. I waved frantically to get his attention above the noise of the saw.

"It's too dangerous for you to be doing that right now. Please come down."

Don straddled a limb. The chain saw dangled from a rope beside him. "It's fire season and these trees need the deadwood cut out," he shouted. "Who else is going to do this? You're not, that's for damn sure." He started the chain saw again.

"So why didn't the doctors say anything? They saw the way I was," Don had said when I'd told him we needed to find a psychiatrist to help him. Our world had become out-of-focus—devoid of the colorful nuances. I couldn't change him, and I couldn't leave him. My days were spent reacting to Don.

Don's strength finally returned—prednisone was working in that regard. He was sleeping better as well due to the Ambien. Don had been working like a fiend with his tree trimming, weed cutting, and hauling of brush on our five acres of property. I helped occasionally, but it was over one hundred degrees many days, and I thought that the tasks were futile. We had hundreds of oak trees on our property. How would clearing a little brush stop a raging fire?

Our wedding anniversary was in August. Although I knew it wouldn't be like old times, we decided to travel to the Southwest for some bike riding. I thought it would be the diversion Don needed from the incessant clearing.

"Didn't Dr. Major say that bike riding was good for you?"

Don looked up from his book. He'd been complaining about needing a break from the clearing. "Yeah, I could time myself to see how my breathing is improving."

We camped the first night near Las Vegas and rode our mountain bikes through Red Rock Canyon. Don took the twelve-mile ride easily, gleefully passing me on every downhill and pumping up the hills to increase his lead. "I haven't felt this good in three months," he told me. We watched shooting stars that night and laughed about the glitz of Las Vegas. The lights were so bright, they obliterated the night sky.

"Look at what all those people are missing," Don said. "Instead of that phony show, they could be watching the real thing right in their backyard."

But two days later, on the morning of our anniversary, Don complained that his hands were cramping, and he didn't want to go outside for the bike ride we had planned near Chaco Canyon. "Why don't you try running hot water on your hands? It's helped before," I suggested. It still felt surreal that his mood had changed so dramatically. He never would have let something like this stop him from doing a sporting activity. Besides using his cane to play tennis, I remember him skiing with a broken hand. He managed to duct tape the pole to his cast.

Don threw down the book he'd been reading. "You just don't get it. You really have no idea what's going on with me. We should have split up years ago." He walked out and drove away, and I didn't see him for the rest of the day.

I began doubting myself. What did he mean when he said we should have split up years ago? I couldn't think of any particular incident or time period he could be referring to. I wasn't perfect. I could be as stubborn as Don and not quick to apologize. Had I falsely believed that we were growing closer again after Don's transplant? Was prednisone the culprit or was there some truth to the comment?

A familiar feeling from childhood gnawed at me. The fear of abandonment. I grew up in a dysfunctional family environment, often afraid that my parents would divorce. They finally did, but not until I went away to college. Between those years I kept hoping things would get better. That my verbally abusive father would change somehow and love my mother again, and that we'd be a family like the Cleavers in *Leave It to Beaver*.

There was always an edge to my father. He could be loving or a brutal totalitarian if angered by some often trivial act. I was highly fearful of his temper. I remember wetting my pants around seven years old when he yelled at me. I don't remember what I did except be in the wrong place at the wrong time. He was cruel and verbally abusive to my mother on many occasions. I never knew my father well enough to know why he was like this. I remember the great relief when I went away to UCLA.

The terrible feeling of insecurity mostly arose during the interactions between my father and mother. She tried sometimes to fight back but didn't have the strength to meet his level of vicious intelligence. When his anger exploded, she would leave the room in tears.

When my parents built an extra wing on the house, my father moved into the new bedroom. It was a turning point for me. We were not going to ever be like the Cleavers. No other kids I knew had parents who slept in separate bedrooms. To me, it signaled something profoundly wrong in my parents' relationship.

It was the same kind of feeling I felt now with Don.

Don didn't speak to me for days, and he only glared when I asked him what was going on. The drive back to California was quiet except for Don's angry outbursts at other drivers, which made me cringe, but I said nothing. I built a wall around myself, pretending that we were two unrelated people sharing the same house. It felt like I'd never known him.

Except for the hand-cramping, Don had seemed better physically. If I stayed with him, I'd have to accept a different kind of marriage, one which was centered on him and this new personality, instead of us. I'd have to get used to waking up every day wondering what the new normal might be and downplaying signs that things might be headed for a major calamity. How long could this last?

He had never been like this. Was it possible that the prednisone was permanently affecting him? Since Don adamantly refused to get psychiatric help and my suggestions only triggered a torrent of verbal abuse, I had to get his doctors to help. Don listened to them and respected them, yet they were more concerned with his physical survival.

In the coming weeks, Don continued to recover physically. His prednisone dose was still high at 90 milligrams a day. Don had been on it for so long and at such a high dose that he had to be tapered off or risk nausea, diarrhea, extreme fatigue, and joint pain.

Around this time, his mood changed. His old enthusiasm returned along with a creative drive. Unfortunately, his attitude toward me became worse—malevolent. He began to attack me in a new way: financially. I noticed that Don had taken forty thousand dollars out of our banking account. I confronted him when he got home from his early morning tennis game. "What did you do with this money?"

"I opened another account in my name," he said. "I'm tired of asking you before I buy something, and I need it to buy another house Sue Wray has lined up for me. Besides, it's the money my mother left me." He smiled slyly. "And the houses I bought in Ohio are all in my name, so you can't get your hands on the rent checks."

I couldn't believe this was actually Don, my savior and teammate.

"So this is the way it is now—*your* money, *my* money? I guess I need to open my own account."

Don slammed the glass he'd been holding down on the counter and it shattered in his hand. He smiled grimly and swept up the shards with a whisk broom. I realized that I'd have to be secretive about my plans in the future. Don was capable of financially destroying me.

It was like playing chess as I considered all the counter moves I could take to safeguard my money. We used my pension check to pay most of our bills, and there was little left at the end of the month. Don's pension check was meager since he'd retired early after his cancer diagnosis. We had a small emergency fund, but that wouldn't last long. We were financially bound, if not emotionally. Neither of us could afford to live separately, even if we sold the house.

This glum insight into what the future held for me was chilling. An older woman "of a certain age" living alone. I saw myself through a distorted lens, not realizing how unfocused the image was. Prednisone was a cruel filter.

What I'd always admired about Don was his courage and determination. During the aftermath of his bone marrow transplant the nerves in his legs were affected, and he couldn't play tennis, a sport he loved. But he became the talk of the courts when he began playing with a cane—managing to compensate for his lack of a backhand by some fast shuffling.

He had been my first love, and, for over forty years, he was perfect in my eyes. He took his responsibilities very seriously, including his defense of me against anyone who showed me disrespect. During our first year of marriage, I was fired as a hostess after only one day on the job and no training. When I came home in tears, Don went to the restaurant and lambasted the manager so ferociously the man threatened to call the police.

It seemed like these personality traits had been exaggerated so outlandishly, making him a caricature of his normal self. Gone was the patience he displayed when showing me how to get out of a riptide by not struggling against it. He tried to teach me to surf, ski, and play tennis, but I didn't have the drive to get beyond the awkward learning phases of those sports, and I gave up on all of them.

Memories of my loving relationship eventually faded completely as the prednisone continued to alter Don's brain. One day I opened a letter from our insurance company. Don had apparently called to have me removed as his beneficiary, and the letter stated that I would have to sign an agreement first to verify that I agreed with the decision.

After forty-two years of mutual sharing of all things, it was impossible to believe that he would delete me as the beneficiary on his life insurance. If he could do this, what else was he capable of?

I showed him the letter. "Why did you do this? Do you hate me so much?"

"I don't trust you. You've been acting so secretive. I think you're planning to leave me."

"I can't believe it's come to this. That you would actually go this far to hurt me."

Don looked embarrassed, which surprised me. "It doesn't matter if you don't sign it." He tore the letter up.

"Please see a psychiatrist," I said. "You're so angry all the time, and you can't control your temper. You've never been this bad before on prednisone. Why don't you talk to your doctors? There must be something you can take or maybe they can refer you to someone who can evaluate you." Don had been a school psychologist and a counselor at a halfway house, and he was a believer in the power of therapy. But his argument was different than what I expected.

Don turned rigid. "There's nothing wrong with me. If you'd gone through what I have, you'd be pissed off too."

Few people *had* gone through his pain and near-death experiences. Over the past ten years, he'd nearly died of leukemia, graft-versus-host disease, and a virulent skin cancer that took his ear and chewed up the right side of his face.

"It's you who has the problem," he ranted. "You're the one causing me to act this way. If you'd just stop bothering me I'd be fine."

But Don's rage extended to anyone who crossed him, especially those who confronted him. I overheard him talking loudly on the phone to his brother about an altercation he had in a bar in Ohio. "I was asking this guy in a bar if he knew of any young men looking for work who could help me fix up houses, and out of nowhere he says, 'I know the real reason you're looking for young guys.' Can you believe that? The asshole was actually calling me a pervert. I demanded that he apologize, and when he didn't I picked up my empty beer bottle and smashed it against the table. You should have seen the fucker's eyes when I held that broken bottle over his head."

I couldn't imagine it. I knew he could be intimidating. He'd always been a man of action, rarely backing down from a confrontation if he was right. He'd stood up to bosses and authority figures before, but bar fights were not his style. In fact, he rarely drank, and he hardly ever agreed to go to a bar. "It's just a scene for loners and losers," he said.

There was no way I could force him to see a psychiatrist. There was a way I could have him hospitalized in a psychiatric ward for seventy-two hours, but Don could seem normal, especially if it suited him. He'd charm the medical staff into releasing him after three days, angrier at me because of my betrayal.

His doctors were the only way. I could appeal to Dr. Massie, his local oncologist, and he might be able to give me advice or have Don hospitalized. I'd learned that the only way someone could be involuntarily hospitalized was if they were a danger to themselves or others. I contacted Dr. Massie's office. It was very difficult to say the words, but I thought they'd trigger the quickest response, "It's urgent that I talk to Dr. Massie right away," I told the receptionist the words I'd rehearsed, but it was still difficult to say: "Don is a danger to himself and others."

I expected the words would push a button prompting immediate action from the authorities. I waited for two days but Dr. Massie never returned my call. I called again and asked if he got the message, and was told that yes, the doctor had read it. Don had an upcoming appointment. Maybe Dr. Massie was waiting to see Don and he'd react to my message then?

Don went to his appointment and came home laughing, "I was in and out of there in five minutes. Dr. Massie said the lab reports looked great."

My words meant nothing. He must have read my note about Don being a danger to himself or others.

"Did Dr. Massie talk to you about anything else?"

"He just asked when I was going back up to Maynard. He was really busy with lots of patients to see."

Since Dr. Massie had ignored my request to speak to him, I had to get help from Don's other doctors. He had an appointment at Maynard coming up with both of them. It was time to insist. If I told them how bad things were, they would surely intervene to get Don psychologically evaluated.

Later, when I recalled Don's behavior to my own psychiatrists, they were shocked that Don had not been treated for his mental illness. "Your husband should have been under psychiatric care," they said. "Any doctor should know what such high a dose of prednisone can do."

I knew that Don's doctors were doing what they could to save his life. They just didn't understand about how mentally ill he was. Like many experts in the medical field, they didn't perceive prednisone for the serious threat it was. They were quick to treat all the other side effects: diabetes, high blood pressure, ulcers, perforation of the bowel, susceptibility to viral, fungal, and parasitic infections, and osteoporosis.

I ran various scenarios about how I'd describe Don's behavior to make the strongest case for immediate psychological intervention. I couldn't see myself pointing to Don in front of his doctors and saying, "He's a danger to himself and others," and those fateful words hadn't prompted any action before. I had to figure out how to talk to the doctors without Don being present. I had to be careful or my plan would backfire, and he would make my life even more miserable. If I went with Don, I could pull his doctors aside.

A big mistake I'd made was in not making sure Don's doctors took care of his mental health concerns. I was too easily put off by their authoritative manner. They were considered gods in their fields. They had treated many people with prednisone. They had saved countless lives. Mostly, they genuinely liked Don. He was known as the poster child of the BMT team at Maynard Hospital.

Getting to Maynard was a long road trip from our house in Atascadero, an excruciating six-hour drive when Don was most vulnerable to his rages. I now knew what 'roid rage was. "Fucking asshole," he'd shout if someone wouldn't pull over to let him pass. He had an uncanny intuition about where the Highway Patrol lurked and slowed down before he hit their radar. Don had been the most careful and patient of drivers before.

"You're really scaring me," I said while we sat in a McDonald's parking lot, where we had stopped for coffee. But my plan was to take the wheel. "Why don't I drive?"

"No, you're not assertive and you don't drive fast enough," he said. "You'll make us late."

"Please let me drive." I reached over to move his hands from the steering wheel, but Don brushed me away. I tried to pry his fingers off, but he gripped the wheel and pushed me away.

We struggled, fighting like children, and it would have been funny if it weren't so grim. We had strayed beyond the point of compromise and were operating on a primitive, self-centered level. He had always looked out for me—now he was like a toddler in a tantrum. I knew I couldn't force him out of the driver's seat. I thought he'd feel sorry for me and back down when he saw how upset I was. "I can't drive with you when you're like this."

"Then don't." I could see the anger building in his steroid-infused glare. "I'll do better on my own without you around." He got out, slammed his door, and yanked my suitcase from the trunk.

I got out and picked up my suitcase. "I can't believe you're just leaving me here stranded. You need help."

"Fuck you," he said.

I'd heard Don use that word many times recently, and he had applied it liberally to many situations and several people, including his brother Joe. But, despite the verbal assaults from the past few months, my husband had never directed that word toward me. During our long marriage, our relationship had been sometimes contentious, two independent and stubborn individuals vying for a position of power, but we did not resort to hurling profanities.

But this time, his words triggered a response that came from a primitive part of me. Months dealing with him had brought me to this moment of frustration. My patience was gone. I'd been waiting to tell him what I thought, and I felt it was justified. I wasn't talking to my husband, but to whatever he had become. Still, it came out so wrong.

"Die and go to hell," I replied.

I don't know where those words came from, but they signaled that I'd sunk to a new low. I immediately regretted what I said.

Don said nothing, but I could tell that my words had affected him because the rage was replaced by a dim understanding, an acknowledgment of our plight. I thought that he would muster the control he needed to come back to me—as Don, not this horrifying stand-in. But he walked to the car without looking back, got in the driver's seat, and drove away.

Our fighting had been louder than I thought, and we had attracted attention. People in the parking lot stared at me. One mother who had been approaching with her toddler grabbed his hand and pulled him farther away from me like I was potentially dangerous. I wheeled my suitcase past the kiddie play area down to the sidewalk, leaving the Happy Meals and chorus of normal family life behind.

The vicious cruelty of what I'd said made me realize that I needed therapy myself. My usual method of coping by gritting my teeth and bearing it was ineffective. And trying to meet on his cold and uncaring level did not make me feel like I was standing up for myself. All I'd cared about was driving through the hard shell of Don's psychosis to his core, trying to make him feel the utmost pain.

I hated what I was becoming. His mental illness was dragging me down too, and we were both headed to the darkest places imaginable. After I figured out how to get home, I'd write down all of Don's episodes and I'd call his doctors. It might be easier that way, with Don not in the same room.

I called my daughter, Anna, but she didn't answer. I was a few miles out of town with no taxi or bus service. I tried to strike a purposeful pose when I drew stares from people unused to seeing a woman standing on the curb with a suitcase in their suburban town. I had to ask for help, which meant explaining my circumstances to a friend or relative in some way that sounded plausible without revealing my obviously fractured life. I waved off a few Good Samaritans and a policeman who drove by before Anna finally called me back and came to get me. She knew her father's awful transformation herself and asked no questions.

* * *

I felt helpless. I sensed that Don was in serious danger, but I wasn't expressing it clearly to his doctors. The Maynard doctors had to be told in a way that would make them act on Don's—and my—behalf. I did what I knew best: as a former librarian, I was well acquainted with research. I needed to make my case. I also needed to focus on something to stop the rising panic and feeling of impending doom, my new constant companion. I began researching prednisone's side effects on personality so that I could arm myself for discussions with Don's doctors. I concentrated on research from peer-reviewed journals and psychiatric studies. I wanted to make sure I was getting valid information.

I found plenty of research on prednisone. I was stunned at what I read. Studies discussed symptoms of psychiatric effects of corticosteroids such as prednisone included cognitive, mood, anxiety, and psychotic symptoms.

> Among 122 patients, 40% experienced depression, followed by mania (28%), psychosis (14%), delirium (10%), and mixed mood episodes (8%).

Among 130 patients, mania was most prevalent (35%), followed by depression (28%), mixed mood episodes (12%), delirium (13%), and psychosis (11%).

In a prospective study of 50 patients treated with corticosteroids, 13 developed hypomania and 5 developed depression. (Cerullo 2006)

It was right there in the medical literature: higher and more sustained dosages of prednisone increase severe psychiatric symptoms.

The Boston Collaborative Drug Surveillance Project found the incidence of psychiatric side effects to be about 20 percent in those taking over 80 milligrams a day over more than a few weeks the risk of psychiatric symptoms (Boston Collaborative Drug Surveillance Program 1972).

Don had been taking 90 milligrams a day for at least three months, which placed him at a nearly 20 percent risk for developing psychiatric symptoms. One of the studies even came from the psychiatry department at Maynard Hospital.
Why weren't Don's doctors alarmed by his behavior?
The descriptions of mania and mixed-mood episodes described Don with stunning accuracy, especially his anger and verbal abuse. Now depression was added to the list of psychiatric issues.
By the end of the day I'd read at least fifty articles, dating back to 1990, which warned of the serious mental disturbances caused by prednisone and the importance of patient monitoring on higher doses. It seemed impossible that Don's doctors, especially Dr. Lin, who had regularly prescribed prednisone the past five years, could be unaware of this information. A new insecurity nagged at me: maybe the doctors weren't taking the link to mental illness seriously enough.
My research also led me to other information linking high doses of prednisone to severe *psychiatric disturbances*. A report published in the Mayo Clinic mentioned that while mania is the most frequent response to the use of steroids, depression is often triggered

by steroid withdrawal (Warrington and Bostwick 2006). There was so much documentation, so many warnings.

Dr. Lin had treated Don since 2007 and had advocated for his bone marrow transplant. She was brilliant, warm, and approachable. Don regarded her as his friend and savior. I felt I knew her well, and I thought we had operated as a team, routing Don through his many challenges after the bone marrow transplant. She would come to his aid, as she had when he had been hospitalized for GVHD and prednisone psychosis in the past. Dr. Lin had been seeing Don since then and had referred to that episode many times, saying, "No one could have survived what you did."

I called Dr. Lin in the morning prepared to leave a message. She'd help again once I explained Don's symptoms. Miraculously she was in the clinic. I got her on the phone right after she'd seen Don for his appointment.

"Something is seriously wrong with Don since you increased his prednisone. First, he was manic. Now he's violent and irrational. He nearly got into a fight in a bar. I'm afraid he's going to hurt someone."

I continued at a controlled pace, trying to appeal to her professional sensibilities by sounding thoughtful and self-confident, not emotional and distressed. I tried to paint an accurate picture of Don by using words I'd read in the research that describe a bipolar person: "manic," "pressured speech," "violent rages," "throwing things," "abusive," "irrational," "road rage," "in serious need of psychiatric help." I stopped short of saying I couldn't tolerate being around him anymore and that our relationship had crumbled. Our personal life wasn't her problem.

Dr. Lin had filtered out the words that should have raised a red flag. There was no alarm in her tone. "Yes, I told him when I saw him today that if I didn't know him, I'd think he was scary. I heard he had an altercation with a parking attendant when he arrived for his appointment. I'm going to taper him off prednisone." Slow tapering was required, meaning it would take several weeks to reduce Don's current dosage of 100 milligrams, and for the psychotic symptoms to subside.

I'd hoped that she would bring up drug treatments like lithium or other psychotropic drugs the articles had mentioned since she had noticed his condition and said he'd been scary, but she didn't seem very concerned. I didn't think I could wait several weeks for Don to recover. What options did I have? My sister lived three hours away, Don's brother lived nearby, and a friend I'd confided in had invited me to stay with her. But I didn't want to admit to anyone about the horror my life had become. And I was embarrassed to hide out like an abused wife.

"Tapering will take a while before Don is normal again," I implored her, trying not to sound desperate. "Can you at least call in a psychiatrist or give Don some kind of medication to help? He is not in control of himself."

"No, Don will be fine once we taper him off," she said firmly. "We're giving him Advair instead." Advair was an inhalant prescribed for people with chronic pulmonary disease like what Don was currently experiencing.

"But what about the next time he gets GVHD again? He's been on prednisone for his skin, his liver, and his eyes. Advair will only work on the pneumonia."

"It's been six years since he had the bone marrow transplant, and GVHD usually doesn't recur after that." I sensed that Dr. Lin thought I was exaggerating, that I wanted Don on drugs for selfish reasons because he was difficult to live with. She insisted that Don would not have to be on prednisone again. She seemed so sure, but I was not convinced. It was as if she'd discounted what I'd said.

Don also had an appointment with Dr. Major that day, so I emailed him. He and Don had chatted about tennis and bicycling at previous appointments. Dr. Major had even given Don his personal cell phone number when we were in Ohio so that he could monitor Don's condition more closely.

I chose my words carefully, for maximum effect. "Don has become out of control. He is manic and violent with terrible episodes of verbal abuse and road rage. He needs psychiatric help. Since you are seeing him today, can you prescribe psychotropic drugs?"

Dr. Major sent me back a cryptic email: "I don't want to put Don on drugs."

"Why not?" I emailed back.

"Sometimes it makes the mental illness worse."

In the few months it would take to taper Don off the drug, I would not be able to escape. I'd been certain that Don would get treatment and, instead, he was being sent back to me in the same state, probably angrier at me for "reporting" on his behavior to his doctors.

I felt abandoned by the doctors. Not only had they refused to treat Don's psychosis themselves, they had refused to refer him to a psychiatrist. Both doctors failed to understand how serious Don's mental illness was.

* * *

Don returned from Maynard saying nothing about his visit other than, "I'm going to get that parking attendant who wouldn't let me park in the drop-off zone so that I could make my appointment. I'm going to write out a complaint and have that motherfucker fired."

"Did Dr. Lin see you like this?"

"Yeah, I was mad. I had her call the guy's supervisor." Then Don laughed. "After I told her she said, 'You know, if I didn't know you, I'd think you were scary.'"

While I waited for the prednisone to release its grip on Don, I continued plodding along with blind faith in the doctors and their assurances that a return to normality was imminent. If no one was going to tell me what was wrong with Don, I would diagnose him myself. My research led me to conclude that Don's symptoms were similar to those described for bipolar disorder.

What was I going to do with this knowledge? I couldn't go to the police. There is no law against being bipolar. I couldn't check him in to a hospital unless he agreed to go, which he had already refused to do. I carried on as if my life was normal. Don had to be tapered at 5 milligrams a week, a grindingly slow pace.

I tried to endure Don, but he kept hammering nails in our relationship.

The summer of 2013 dragged on and I watched and waited, spending most of my time inside to avoid the oppressive heat. As Don came and went, my vision narrowed to my immediate surroundings. I focused on incremental changes in my environment. I watched birds build their nests and raise multiple broods. The nests had to be inaccessible or the blue jays would find them and kill the young. A pair of vireos with smoky-colored circles around their eyes built a nest on a ledge under the rafters, outside my kitchen window. Their nests were small and neat, like woven baskets. They kept them clean by removing the droppings and food remnants. The finches made big, sloppy nests from weeds and needle grass, which they scavenged from the ground, and took no care to accurately shape. The deck below was littered with debris that didn't make it to the nest. The nest itself and surrounding area was covered with bird shit, which hardened like cement and was difficult to wash off. I kept watch at my kitchen window, and if I saw them trying to construct their nest, I had to move quickly, before they laid their eggs, and sweep it away with a broom.

In retaliation, the house finches ganged up on my precious vireos and pushed their nest off the ledge onto the deck. So strong and well-constructed, it maintained its perfect form next to the scattered mess of the house finches. The vireo pair had been bullied away by the finches and retreated to an oak tree to watch the destruction. I picked up the nest and put it back in the same spot, but the vireos never returned to reclaim it.

Chapter 4
Respite

Finally, I began noticing a change in Don's mood after six weeks. I was cautiously optimistic. I hadn't seen Don in a rage for about a week, but I was still suspicious that I might unintentionally provoke him.

One morning, he backed into the garage door before it opened completely and blamed it on me. "This is your fault," he raged as he hammered at the bent and damaged door that was stuck halfway down. "You distracted me. You know you did." My crime: I'd run out of the house while he was backing out and asked him when we were dropping off my car at the shop.

After a few minutes of ferocious banging he backed off and apologized. "I know it wasn't your fault. I was just pissed off at myself. How could I have not realized the door wasn't completely open?" He pushed the switch and the motor whirred, but the door only went up a foot before it jammed. He shook his head and began rummaging in his tool chest, extracting an enormous screw driver.

"Why don't I call the company to repair it?" I thought of him blundering around, making things worse.

"No, let me try it out first." He carefully examined the door. "I think it's just bent a little right here." Don used the screwdriver as a wedge to straighten out the metal. He pushed the remote and the door jittered up and down the track. "So, what do you think? Am I better?"

The fix was only temporary, but I laughed at his eagerness to hear a compliment from me. A month ago, on 90 milligrams, he would have worked out his frustration by hammering the door into submission or damaging it beyond repair. The tapering seemed to be working. I was noticing small yet significant signs of improvement.

That night I allowed myself to feel optimistic, that hope was on the horizon. It was a brilliant night full of promise and reflection.

Jill Stegman

An asteroid display was supposed to be seen in the early morning hours.

I was watching a TV series, *Breaking Bad*, which friends had recommended. They said Don reminded them of the lead character, Walter White, the same seamed face and beard, his intelligence and courage. Don had been a teacher, and he did resemble Walter in terms of his "take no prisoners" attitude. I'd just lived through a lifetime of anxiety these past months, and watching TV had become part of my evening routine. I couldn't concentrate on reading, though it had been one of my life's great pleasures.

Parts of the plot were absurd. What made me keep watching was that, like Walter, Don was canny and smart, and he cared for his family above all else. I was waiting and hoping for his return to the man he had been.

As on many evenings, Don was out on the deck, staring into the black void and probably contemplating whatever random thoughts occurred to him. I usually left him alone out there, happy for the partition of the night.

I knew he could see me inside the well-lit house, but I couldn't see him very well in the dark. We were back-to-back, only separated by the sliding glass door. I couldn't stay interested in Walter's dramatized plight with my own plight so vividly nearby. His slow return to normalcy made me want to join Don and be in his presence even if we said nothing to each other. I turned off the TV and went outside.

Don was gazing at the star-littered sky when I pulled up a chair to sit beside him. "What are you thinking about?"

He pointed out to the horizon. "I'm tracing the planes coming in from the east and figuring out which airport they're headed to." We lived between San Francisco and Los Angeles, so planes coming from the east flew over us before splitting north or south. I'd noticed it before, but I was happy to hear Don explaining something in his patient teacher-voice. Some planes didn't veer north or south, but headed directly west, eventually seeming to disappear over the ocean at a certain point. It was a curious phenomenon that I didn't completely understand.

"Does it have to do with the curvature of the Earth?" I didn't care if he was condescending and acted like I was one of his eighth-grade students. I'd be happy if he showed me how to tie my shoelaces, as long as he talked to me.

"That's somewhat true," he said, laughing at my simplistic explanation. "But it probably has more to do with the vanishing point. Since the airplane is traveling parallel to the earth, both will eventually meet at some point on the horizon."

We watched the planes and their trajectories for hours, spotting shooting stars and satellites beeping across at higher levels. We tried to guess constellations, although I could only locate the Big Dipper. Don pointed out how some planets formed part of the constellations. His explanations helped me see the sky in a way I'd never noticed before, as a living force. He was so animated when he talked.

I couldn't see his face clearly in the dark, but his voice had lost the weirdly pressured tone. To me this signaled that Don was coming back. He was at a turning point, and able to focus again. He'd been adrift for so long, it must have felt like regaining consciousness. And I was with him. I could have lingered there all night just listening to his voice.

The next morning Don spent more time on the computer writing his memoir while I went back to revising my novel. I read some of Don's memoir; he'd been working on it for about five years, mostly when he was on prednisone and had the fire in him. I hadn't read any of it recently, and I was impressed by his insight and reflections. How he wanted to inspire others with cancer. It had to be a positive sign of recovery.

> In the last eleven years, I have been told that I had two years to live. I have a bone marrow transplant. My new bone marrow has attacked parts of my body three times with GVHD. I have had fifty-plus blood transfusions, thirty days of radiation, thirty days of chemotherapy. I have no ear or hair on one side of my head. I have lost some of my salivary glands. I have lost and regained my sense of taste, had hepatitis-like conditions twice, temporary diabetes twice, nerve damage to my right side, damage to my right eye, and have some pretty long surgical scars from the top of my skull to the carotid artery on my neck, I need an artificial knee, but I can live with this . . . emphasis on the word "live." *I am still fighting medical problems and anticipate that this battle will end only when something gets me before I get rid of it.*

As I write this book, I am currently being treated for a rare type of pneumonia (COP), so recently renamed that my own family physician hadn't even heard the new name given to the disease. I have a knee replacement scheduled for a month from now. Again, I say life is good. I embrace it and I have learned that I am much stronger in spirit and body than I ever thought possible eleven years ago. So are you! You are much stronger in mind, body, and spirit than you presently imagine. Your own life strands, how you've faced early and later life challenges, have taught you much more than you currently utilize. If you have been diagnosed with a supposed terminal condition, you have a chance to beat it. You have it in you to beat it. You are capable of pulling together your collective life experiences to use them to fight what initially seem unconquerable.

I am proof that such a statement can be true. I am not the only survivor of so called "terminal conditions" to make such statements. This book is meant to encourage, inform, and sometimes entertain you. Life is the unexpected/tough/funny/good/sad/challenging/_____ (you fill in your adjectives). Life has more dimensions once you've faced very difficult problems. You have a choice. Fight hard to not give in to feelings of helplessness and hopelessness. You are someone who can make it. Set your mind to that. You'll come out the other end of your condition discovering how resilient you really are.

* * *

We planned a trip to Lake Tahoe for bike riding and hiking. Don had recovered enough from the pneumonia and was ready to test his state of fitness in the higher altitude of the mountains. The setting was clear and pristine. It was October, the so-called shoulder season because the summer visitors had left, and the dropping temperatures anticipated winter. We stayed at the Olympic Village Inn, a faux-chalet–style motel in Squaw Valley where Don had tried to teach me to ski forty-some years ago on our first anniversary. Don was a patient teacher, trying to point out a visual for me to sight before moving my skis cautiously from one spot to the next. But I'd proven to be lead-footed, as awkward as a penguin out of water. I couldn't let my body relax like Don could. I felt out of control when my skis slid on the snow, and it threw me into a panic, followed by the proverbial face-plant. When we rode up the ski lift after a run, I wished I were one of the workers helping people off.

We rode our bikes along the Truckee River, Don timing his rides to note improvement in his lung capacity. Although he wasn't in perfect health, he had improved dramatically from Ohio. But something was different. His rage was gone for the most part, yet he wasn't fully Don. I kept waiting for the resilient charge of his personality to return showing *he was back*. Instead I sensed that he was going through the motions of what was expected, but his heart wasn't in it. He'd ridden ahead and I found him by the side of a trail, staring at the river washing through Squaw Valley. The aspens were dropping their leaves and some of them twirled in the water. I pulled my bike over to Don. He was wearing his hat with the shade screen. He looked slumped and beaten.

"How are you doing? Are you enjoying this?" I said.

He picked up a small rock and examined it. "It's fine."

"Is the altitude getting to you? Is that why you stopped?" We were at eight thousand feet above sea level.

He threw the pebble at one of the leaves floating by. "No, it isn't the altitude. I'm just tired. Nothing seems like that much fun anymore."

I didn't know what to say so I gave him my usual pep talk that sounded trite even to me after so many repetitions. "But you're so much better." I hugged him. "I love being here with you."

I decided it wasn't anything to worry about. I mistook a dampening of spirit for inward reflection. Who could imagine how it felt to return from madness to a sense of control? Of course, it would take time for him to fully return to his old self. I convinced myself it was just a matter of patience.

Things were calm over the next few days. It snowed one morning, just lightly enough to melt soon after falling, just enough to signal the transition to winter. We started off in heavier jackets and long pants and shed that gear by noon, feeling like bears coming out of hibernation. You'd never have known that winter was at the back door and the bike paths would soon be covered with snow until spring.

Don got frustrated trying to mount the bikes on the car rack. He wasn't as strong as he used to be, and the mountain bikes were heavy and awkward. Instead of walking away from the swearing and furor, I offered to help.

Don started to react like he usually did in these circumstances. "And what exactly can you do? If I can't lift these motherfuckers up, how can you?"

It was cold outside, the temperature was dropping again since we got back from the bike ride, and Don's fingers and hands had to be freezing. I wasn't going to leave him alone. The trip wasn't going to end like this.

I made a stab at what I knew was a feeble suggestion. "I'll stay out here with you in case I can do something."

Don shook his head, mumbling about "stupid, half-assed plans."

"Maybe I can lift the bikes up to you while you hoist them up?"

Don opened the car door and stood on the door jam, "I don't think you're strong enough for this, but let's try it out. Don't do anything until I tell you to. I don't want to drop the bike."

"Your wish is my command."

I lifted the front part of the bike by the handlebars and Don grabbed it, pulling it up. Then I moved to the seat and rear tire balancing the bulk over my head while Don positioned it on the rack. "Move it left," "Grab the frame," or "Hold it steady, dammit!" Finally, Don secured it in place and locked it down.

"High fives," I said, reaching up to slap his palm. "So, did I help?"

Don looked down at me, amused. "Yeah," he chuckled. "I'd hire you." I caught a glimpse of the man I knew. We both blew on our hands to warm them up to load the other bike. He winced as if trying to tackle an unsettling thought, trying to move it to the back of his mind. "It was good having you out here with me."

I thought this was a sign of good things to come. I magnified the event way out of proportion—not understanding the dips and plateaus of depression and the constant nagging of doubt even in the face of what life has to offer.

* * *

Don was quieter, but his silence was furtive rather than peaceful. He spent more time at the computer and quickly closed whatever he was working on if I came into the room. I thought it was strange when he insisted on setting himself up as a separate user with a password—we had always shared the same email account. I wasn't too concerned because we had already resolved the financial crisis. Don put my name on the bank account he'd opened, and I was no longer worried that he was plotting against me. We'd already received the first payment from the rental houses in Ohio, and the toll it had taken on our lives was a faraway nightmare.

In the last weeks of October 2013, when Don occasionally got frustrated, I did my best to soothe him. He was down to 10 milligrams. One morning I went for a walk while Don did his usual morning session inhaling Advair through a tubular attachment on his nebulizer, a small machine that resembled a humidifier. Don had to use the nebulizer morning and night to control the pneumonia. He often grumbled about feeling "like an addict needing a fix," but realized its importance to his recovery. But this time, he became enraged at the machine for some reason. I returned to a scene of chaos, Don shouting, "Goddamn it!" He pointed to the shattered nebulizer lying on the bathroom floor. "That cheap-ass bastard wasn't working right."

I picked up the badly cracked machine. "Maybe we can get it to work until we can buy you another one." I tried to patch it back together with Don's medical tape, but it only emitted a strangled gasp when we turned it on. We both realized what it meant to lose this machine that was Don's lifeline.

I assumed my "take-charge" role, one that I'd been so good at before. "I'll order another one from the internet." I retrieved my laptop and began browsing the manufacturer's website while Don paced angrily, which I tried to ignore. I wanted so much to show him I could "fix" things, even if I couldn't actually make the repairs.

I found the image of Don's specific machine on the site and paid just about as much as the nebulizer cost for overnight shipping. "We'll get it tomorrow. It's guaranteed one-day delivery."

This was what I was good at, trying to make things better. It was a mode of interacting that had worked so well seven years ago, when Don was recovering from his bone marrow transplant. I exaggerated this one small success so much I missed the warning in the flatness of Don's response. He wasn't nearly as excited as I was. "Great," was all he said.

I looked forward to Don's next appointment with Dr. Major. I was sure Don would show improvement, and that his lungs would be clear of the ominous gray film that had showed up in the last X-rays. I'd forgiven Dr. Major for not treating Don's psychosis, because I was flush with the warm wash of relief that Don had conquered yet another threat to his health. This was just the news Don needed to jolt him out of his despondency. Everything would be fine. Don would recover and his spirits would pick up. He would find joy and excitement in life again.

Don made his rounds at the clinic, first doing the labs for his blood work, then on to two different X-rays of his lungs. As usual, the reception area and waiting rooms were full of sick people in various stages of treatment for cancer and life-threatening diseases. Some hobbled on canes and walkers. Many with compromised immune systems wore respirators that looked like gas masks, their eyes desperate and fearful, which must have seemed depressing to the inexperienced visitor. To me it was a sign of hope to contrast Don with the other patients at their various stages of treatment. His appearance had changed, and he was missing his right ear, but he wore his scars like a warrior's badges. Writing his memoir had demonstrated how strong he felt with what he had lived through, and he was eager to share his experiences.

We ate lunch outside by the pond, watching a female mallard with her new brood. We had watched her raise her offspring each time we visited. It didn't occur to me that it might not be the same duck we had observed over the past seven years.

The usually severe-looking Dr. Major smiled when he flipped Don's charts up on the monitor, showing that Don's lungs were 95 percent back to full capacity. "This is a better recovery than I ever expected."

I was waiting for Don to react to the good news, but there was no sign that his spirits had been lifted. He seemed dazed, as if the full impact had not hit him. "So, does that mean I can get off the nebulizer?"

Dr. Major looked surprised by Don's blunted reaction. "No, we'll have to keep you on that for some time."

"How long?"

"I can't say right now. We want to make sure you're not going to relapse."

Don didn't say anything, but I saw that he was disturbed by what Dr. Major said. The good news of his recovery should have overwhelmed the fact that he had to stay on the nebulizer.

"We should go celebrate," I said on our way back to the car.

"Why? I hate the damn nebulizer. I can't stand to think I'll be sucking on that thing twice a day indefinitely."

"This doesn't sound like the normal way you receive good news about your health. You should be elated. You just beat something else. At least you're not on oxygen."

"It's been seven goddamned years, and I'm still on drugs. My goal was to be drug-free by now, but something else keeps coming up, and I don't want to be on prednisone again."

Don's tone worried me. He seemed resigned and defeated.

"I talked to Dr. Lin. She said you wouldn't have to be on it again." Even as I said this, I realized that we both knew that Dr. Lin couldn't predict the future.

"No." Don shook his head as if he'd made up his mind about something.

Don turned inward during the next few weeks. He performed his daily routines in a robotic manner. He usually came back from tennis elated and charged with the competition, but now he seemed not to get the same enjoyment from the sport he'd loved for over twenty-five years. The high energy with which he usually described his tennis game was replaced with a shrug of indifference. "It was OK."

I wasn't too concerned, because I was looking for depression like I'd seen before when he refused to get out of bed.

Now, Don kept asking, "Am I better?"

"Yes, so much better." But I saw a lost look in his eyes like he was fighting something.

"I just feel so guilty for the way I was."

"Don't worry. I'm already forgetting it. It's over and we're going back to the way we were." And I believed these words as I said them.

Prednisone was slowly releasing its grip on Don. It was just a matter of time before he returned to normal.

For now, I would accept Don's current state. Anything was better than the anxiety and chaos I'd lived through. Our relationship was no longer a flaming asteroid on a collision course destroying everything in its path. This was only a phase of adjustment as we returned to our routines.

I was writing again in the morning, making hesitant progress on my novel, absorbed in my characters. Don came and went during the time I wrote, and we were a couple in the afternoons. He was still quiet, but I told myself that he was just being reflective. He must have been torn up by the anguish and horror of the forces that had been at work to destroy him.

I didn't even think it was strange when Don became obsessed about me not driving the truck. I attributed it to a quirkiness of his along the twisted path to recovery. He asked me every time he went out if I was planning on going somewhere. If I was, he drove the truck to be sure I drove the car. I had put a few dents in the truck, and didn't like driving it, so I assumed Don was trying to be thoughtful.

One day I decided to go to the library to research an aspect of my novel, but Don had already taken the car. When I climbed behind the wheel of the truck, I noticed a strange bundle in the backseat. Don had taken a canvas bag from our sleeping bag and stuffed something inside that looked like a rifle. I thought it might have been my son's old BB gun because I'd hidden the rifle and the shotgun when Don was so violent. But he had changed so dramatically from the former irrational version of himself, I didn't consider him capable of shooting someone or of any act of violence.

Don was pacing in the garage when I returned. "Why didn't you tell me you were going somewhere when I asked you this morning?"

I thought his concern was a little exaggerated. "I changed my mind and drove the truck, and now I'm back safe and sound." I walked past him.

Don followed me into the house. "You need to make sure you tell me from now on."

"What's the big deal? Why don't you want me to drive the truck?"

"I think there might be something wrong with the brakes."

"If there's something wrong, we should take the car to the shop."

"Yeah," he said. "I'll take care of it. In the meantime, don't drive it."

I would forget about what I had seen in the backseat until much later, when it was too late and all that was left to do was obsess over trying to put the puzzle pieces together.

* * *

Don began disappearing for periods of time, not saying where he was going. He'd come back in two hours to go on a bike ride or walk on the beach. It was wonderful grabbing his hand as we took in the cool breeze. He always checked the tides first so that the low tide left a wide swath of packed sand to walk on. He was still paranoid of getting skin cancer again, so he wore a French Foreign Legion–style hat with a drape attached to cover his neck. A neighbor woman saw him walking with this hat once and asked him if he was a Muslim because, in her uneducated view, the hat looked like a keffiyeh, worn by Arab men. We later laughed when we found out that she had thought Don might be a terrorist on the run.

One day Don disappeared for several hours, and he came back unusually excited, wanting to talk about his drive. He had been at Whale Rock Reservoir, an unspectacular hillside above the ocean with a fabulous view where we often rode our bikes. I'd never known Don to be particularly fond of the place, but I was happy it had triggered such a positive reaction.

"Let's go for a walk on the beach tomorrow and have lunch in Cayucos," he said. Cayucos was a beach town near Whale Rock Reservoir. We liked it for its casual lack of pretension, where it was hard to detect the locals from the tourists. Its vibe never evolved from the sixties, though the houses had increased in value exponentially. Don had taught our children and nephews to surf here while I walked the shoreline.

Don still maintained his upbeat tone the next day. It was as if something had lifted and a new light shone through. When we got to the beach, the tide had brought in small, harmless jelly-fish type creatures which sprouted tiny dorsal "sails of membrane" that allowed them to skim across the sea with the wind. Don examined one of them in his palm. "Look at that. They get blown across the sea their whole lives and have to trust that they'll be safe, but they end up tossed ashore and abandoned like flotsam."

We watched a pair of kite sailors skipping over the waves. Don followed them intently as they performed multiple aerobatics surfing the wave crossways and slipping over the crest before it broke and buried them. "I always wanted to do that." He sounded so wistful.

This was coming from a man who had tried and excelled at any sport he was interested in. He'd played varsity football, basketball, baseball, and tennis. He'd run track, surfed, scuba dived, skied, and skateboarded.

I squeezed his arm more tightly. "Why don't you learn now?"

"You can't do everything. I surfed, and that gave me knowledge of the ocean. What they're doing is something I would have liked, but not now." He glanced away, examining his thoughts. His scar, the "battle wound" he usually wore proudly, looked like a red slash. "I have to tell you something." His face was still drawn and tired. Thankfully he was down to 5 milligrams three times a week and would soon be off prednisone entirely. "I'm really worried about what I've been thinking, but I've been afraid to tell you."

I didn't ask him about his thoughts. If I had I might have acted differently, and my reflection might have exonerated me. Anna and John still can't understand why Don didn't try to get help for himself, especially since he was knowledgeable about mental health. I think John also wonders why I didn't confide to him about Don. When the conversation moves in that direction, John is careful with his words, but when he says, "I wish I'd known that Dad was depressed," I know what is not being said: why didn't you save him?

I knew that Don was looking to me for help. I could have done several things. I could have taken him immediately to an emergency room, I could have called 911 or the Suicide Hotline if I'd realized how serious he was about considering taking his life, but that would have meant fully comprehending the urgency. "I'll call tomorrow and we'll get you to a psychiatrist."

Don nodded, and I thought we were on the right track. He hadn't mentioned the word "suicidal," which would have alerted me to take him to the hospital. I didn't think to question him, or

I would have discovered just how serious his intentions were. He didn't act like he was in imminent danger of harming himself. He had agreed to let me intervene. I was going to get help like before and I would valiantly save him.

One reason why I didn't immediately react to Don's depression was that he had been depressed before, and this time seemed milder in comparison. Six years ago, when we came back to Atascadero after his first diagnosis of prednisone psychosis, I watched him lose interest in everything. He had loved sports of every kind and had never let any ailment hold him back. His competitive presence on the tennis court was well known, even when he once played with a cane. But he became depressed; he refused to go outside and only rode his stationary bike inside, insisting that he would get an infection or a fungal attack outside. When we saw Dr. Lin for Don's monthly appointments, she said depression was normal after a bone marrow transplant. The only advice she gave for his depression was more exercise.

The day came when I could not coax Don out of bed. He lay staring at the ceiling all day, his thrillers scattered, and he admitted he was very depressed. Looking at him in this catatonic state I knew he was barely functioning, suffering from a deep and morbid pain. Dr. Lin was out of the country on one of her many lecture circuits, or she may have been in Tahiti, where she owned a farm. And I'd begun to doubt her prescription of "more exercise" for Don.

I took Don to his old GP, Doctor Long, who diagnosed him as "severely depressed," and prescribed an antidepressant. When we saw Dr. Lin, she said she was happy that Don was doing better and wrote in her notes: "Mr. Stegman was seen by his local GP for depression and was prescribed Celexa."

But this time Don's depression seemed manageable. He wasn't completely bed-ridden like he'd been six years before when he was at Maynard and the first months after we got home. He still functioned and went about his normal activities, even though he didn't enjoy them as much. And he had agreed with me to get help.

That night I emailed Dr. Lin and Dr. Major. "Don has become depressed, and I'm contacting psychiatrists for help."

Dr. Major replied, "Let me know what I can do."

His response struck me as too little too late and lacking. I didn't know what he could do. I needed someone to tell *me* what to do. What I know now is that Don's depression should have alarmed Dr. Major. Some of the reports I read stated that depression was prevalent and very serious during the withdrawal of prednisone. But I didn't know then what I do now. It might not have made a difference if I'd mentioned it to Dr. Major. His cryptic note offered no suggestions. I was on my own.

That night after he had told me he needed help, I was confident that we were on the right track. I would call one of Don's doctors and something would be prescribed. I was giddy with relief thinking of a return to our former state. I kissed Don with a passion I hadn't felt in years, and he'd acted startled at first, stumbling backward like he couldn't believe it was happening—perhaps remembering that only two months ago I'd told him to "die and go to hell." But I'd been trying to make up for those words since his transition.

"What a sweet kiss," he said.

I touched his face. "I want you to know that you're the most important person to me."

Don looked at me in a strange, sad way. "Thank you so much for saying that."

I'd overlooked his odd response and tried to see this gesture as breaking new ground. We'd reached the end of the dark days and were starting a new direction. From now on we would be a force to contend with, a powerful unit representing forty-two years together and surviving the worst trials. A month before I'd wanted Don out of my life, now I couldn't imagine a future without him.

Chapter 5
November 11:
The Devil Takes His Due

While I waited for the doctor's offices to open the morning after Don agreed to get help, I tried to work on my novel. It was the only activity that could distract me. I was on the last chapter, absorbed in wringing the emotional response from the resolution—was the protagonist going to stay in Mexico with his lover or come back to the United States and take on the cartel to exonerate himself?

I thought Don was equally as absorbed with his Ken Follett novel, but mid-morning he abruptly stood up from the table. I hardly paid attention as he rushed into the spare bedroom, grabbed something, and then hurried out to the garage. I heard him start the truck and the grinding of the garage door that he had bashed into earlier. I glanced up when he left, vaguely wondering why he hadn't said where he was going in such a rush.

I tried to continue writing, unsure if I'd reached the end of the novel as I charted a likely course for the protagonist. Suddenly I stopped typing, wondering how long Don had been gone. A cloud of doubt and finality hung in the air overwhelming any interest in writing. Maybe it was only a reminder that I needed to begin contacting Don's doctors. Don had agreed to get help, so he must be planning to return soon.

I called Dr. Massie's office first hoping this was the only call I'd have to make. Dr. Massie was Don's local oncologist, a Maynard affiliate charged with following up with Don after his bone marrow transplant. He had seen Don two months before, after I'd left the note that Don was a danger to himself and others. He'd ignored me then, but now I thought I could get through to him because Don was willing to discuss his depression and cooperate. Massie would prescribe something or send Don to a psychiatrist. When Don returned I'd have an appointment, and we'd laugh at my unfounded anxiety. It was only a matter of getting Don the drugs he needed, and the medical establishment would help as they had before by diagnosing and prescribing the right therapy.

I explained the depression to Dr. Massie's medical assistant in a professional tone, and that I thought it was related to prednisone. She told me that "Dr. Massie does not treat patients for depression or mental issues," and suggested I call a psychiatrist. Which psychiatrist? She had no names for me, "Look at Don's insurance plan to find out who takes his insurance," was her suggestion. I tried my own psychiatrist, Dr. Crosby, who I'd seen once for "general insomnia" issues. A recorded message said she wasn't in the office for a week and suggested calling 911 "if this is an emergency." I called Don's old GP, who had treated him for depression seven years before, but Long was no longer in practice. I called numerous psychiatrists' and psychologists' offices. Either no one was taking new patients or Don would have to wait weeks to be seen.

Hours went by, Don was still not home, and I hadn't gotten any help, nor did anyone seem to want to help. I heard the same mantra over and over, "The doctor is not taking any new patients." I stopped calling when recorded messages told me that offices were now closed for lunch, and I had to return to the stillness of the house.

We had designed and built this house twenty-five years ago. It sat on a hillside in an oak-studded forest overlooking a valley where hawks soared at eye-level. We had envisioned an open, airy home so many years ago when we were planning a life together. A house that would withstand whatever conflicts we might encounter. We'd sat on our deck watching fog banks fingering over the hills from the ocean that blanketed the valley like snow. Nearly every night for twenty-five years, the sunsets had panned the horizon as far as we could see, elaborate pyrotechnical fanfares that consistently drew us outside to observe, arms around each other.

The house was us. We fought and grew apart in this house, but always coming back to each other. Here we raised our children, John and Anna, feeding them on the pleasures of hiking and sharpening their senses to the natural world.

Now I hated being alone here. The walls did not offer safety and security, but harbored confinement and the relentless agony of

November 11: The Devil Takes His Due

waiting for Don's return. I don't know why I didn't call someone—friends or relatives would have offered advice. But I couldn't believe that things were so bad. I had to think I was over-reacting. We had been through a crisis before and emerged triumphantly.

Don and I had planned on going to a movie in the afternoon and I knew he would meet me there. He'd show up smiling, and my worry would dissolve.

I had to do something to pass the time, so I drifted to the computer and started researching prednisone and mental illness, my default anti-anxiety activity. If nothing else, I could learn more about it as ammunition for future appointments with Don's doctors. This time I searched "prednisone and depression," and I was linked to hundreds of websites and reports that led me to a review of the literature in *The American Journal of Psychiatry*:

> Glucocorticoids [including prednisone] increase the risk of suicidal behavior and neuropsychiatric disorders. Educating patients and their families about these adverse events and increasing primary care physicians' awareness about their occurrence should facilitate early monitoring. (Fardet, Petersen and Nazareth, 2012)

What did they mean by "early monitoring?"

> When severe problems with mood, memory, cognition, or behavior occur during glucocorticoid treatment or withdrawal, the prescribing physician should consider consulting with or referring the patient to a knowledgeable psychiatrist . . . Educating patients about possible side effects and the need to report them is essential (Judd et al. 2014).

I stopped reading as a cacophony of voices overcame my last shreds of hope. I next typed in the word *suicide* and found:

> The highest potential for suicide is not necessarily when the person has hit rock-bottom, but when they appear to be getting better. A sudden improvement in mood may indicate the person has made peace with the decision to end their life, and perhaps, even has a plan in place for doing so. As such, if someone has been showing signs of depression, and suddenly seems much happier, you should take preventative steps right away ("How to Recognize the Warning Signs of Suicide" 2018).

Don's excitement at finding Whale Rock Reservoir and his eagerness to take a walk with me! I didn't want to read anymore, but I stared at the next words:

"Those at the highest risk for committing suicide in the near future have a specific suicide PLAN, the MEANS to carry out the plan, a TIME SET for doing it, and an INTENTION to do it."

The means to carry out the plan? The bundle in the back seat I thought looked like a rifle?

Time set for doing it? He's simply driving around, not at Whale Rock Reservoir, where he'd visited yesterday and came home so excited about.

Intention to do it? I'd just told him last night how important he was to me. Don had set the movie date and selected the movie *All Is Lost*. I'd go to the theater and he would be there.

* * *

"I'm not sure where Dad is, but I'm coming home," I had told Anna when she'd called me at the movie theater. "I'll talk to you soon." I wanted so much to add, "It's OK," like I always had before in times of crisis, but I couldn't lie to her. For ten years, the two guns had been casually stashed in the closet with the vacuum cleaner, unloaded and unused, until I moved them. But now there was only one.

I was outside the theater surrounded by people, but I felt ungrounded among them. They were on their way somewhere, but I was directionless, swirling like Robert Redford on a raft in the ocean. Home was the last place I wanted to be. It meant more waiting and admitting that I had to call the police. Don was out there somewhere with a shotgun, and I could have been searching for him, might have saved him. Instead, I spent two hours watching an actor's performance. I had missed the clues. If I'd concentrated, I'd have seen the same look in his eyes as the man at sea: the progression of confidence, resolution, frustration, and the look of resignation at the end.

On the way home, I pulled off the 101 to look at the daytime moon, dimly visible in the eastern sky. Instead of giving me the usual solace of being a part of the larger world, I saw the face of a joker with big, thick lips spread in a jack-o-lantern leer jeering at my Sunday-school inspirations, my missed observations, and my faulty intuitions. For now, I pushed that face away. I had a long night before me.

I had no option but to call the police. Anna was excited to see me until she noticed the look on my face. I paced back and forth from the kitchen to the dining room. "Dad's been gone all day. He's never done anything like this before. I have to call."

"My husband is depressed and he's been gone all day. I don't know where he is," I told the 911 operator. I looked over at Anna. "And I think he has a shotgun with him. It's missing."

"How many hours has he been gone?"

It was now five o'clock. I hadn't noticed the exact time Don left. "It's been about seven hours. He left at around ten this morning."

"You said he was depressed? For how long?"

"I'm not sure how long it's been. He took a drug and it made him psychotic then depressed."

"Has he been this way for days, weeks?"

"He hasn't seemed right for a few weeks, but I didn't know how bad it was until yesterday when he told me that he was afraid of his feelings. Then this morning he drove off."

"Did you see him take the gun?"

By now I was rocking back and forth in the chair as each word drew me closer to the truth. "No, but I saw him grab something out of the bedroom and I know the shotgun is missing now."

"An officer will be there soon."

Officer Garza, young and inexperienced, sat across from Anna and me at the dining room table, stumbling through routine questions in a neutral voice. I tried to recount the details of the past week to create the sense of urgency: the rifle I suspected in the back seat of the truck, Don's weird behavior the day before, and the sickening realization that I suspected he could be at Whale Rock Reservoir, but Garza still got some of the information wrong. I remembered the interview very clearly.

How long has your husband been missing? *Since about ten a.m.*

Did he have a weapon? *Yes, he had a shotgun he must have found after I hid it.*

What was your husband's behavior like recently? Did he seem depressed? *He acted depressed, like he didn't get the same enjoyment out of life, but he got up every day and went about his normal routine. He told me two days ago that he was afraid to tell me his feelings and I got him to agree to seek help. I just started calling for help when he disappeared.*

But the police report read:

"Donald was recently taken off of (prescribed) prednisone and has become 'disconnected' and spends his time in bed. He has admitted to Jill that he feels like 'he has been a burden to the family' and has unfairly dragged them down due to his illness."

I don't know why Sergeant Garza changed what I'd said; he was taking notes. I knew I was trying to create a sense of urgency, but the words he used were not mine. If I'd been an outside observer I would have thought, "Why didn't she get help right away? Why did she wait so long to call when this man was so clearly suicidal?"

Sergeant Garza had completed his questioning. He gave me a reassuring smile. "We'll get on this right away. You know, ninety-nine percent of the time people are found alive."

"But he's been gone all day. What would he be doing that long? He had a shotgun."

"He's probably just sitting somewhere thinking about what's going on in his life."

Officer Garza projected the self-confidence of authority, but the inexperience of youth. I feared that Don had done all his thinking and was succumbing even now to the outcome. By calling the police I'd set the fateful events in motion. I imagined this must be how refugees feel, those who stay behind instead of fleeing a war-torn country, thinking that they are safe against all evidence to the contrary, and then recognizing that they waited too long and are doomed.

I sat on the couch, squeezing Anna's hand as I imagined a team of police officers being immediately dispatched, sirens blaring as they rushed to Whale Rock Reservoir in time to save my husband.

As the hours passed, my house became a prison, and I was captive to my emotions. I felt no comfort sitting among years of accumulated possessions that once had held such significance.

In 1991 a fire had raged across the canyon, and we had evacuated our house for three days. While Anna, John, and our dog, Libby, waited in the car, Don and I grabbed whatever was most important to us. He took the Navajo rug and a few family heirlooms. I picked up the Native American pottery, the hand-blown glass, and the family photo albums.

Now I wanted to burn it all. The house and its familiar objects evoked a past now dead. Sunset, usually my favorite time of day, came and faded quickly—an ugly slash.

* * *

At ten p.m. two officers came to the door. I saw the looks on their faces, standing in the dim light like messengers of doom, their patrol car blinking in the driveway, and I was crying before they even spoke.

"I'm so sorry, but your husband was found dead at Whale Rock Reservoir. He shot himself. I'm so sorry."

"Do I have to identify him?"

"No, he had his ID with him."

Right, he would have thought of that. "Did you find him?"

"No, but I have the name of the person who did. I'm so sorry, Mrs. Stegman." He handed me his card with the case number and the name of the county sheriff who found him.

Anna came up behind me crying, not caring that she was dressed only in a flannel pajama top and lace underwear.

One of the officers gawked at her. "Who's that?"

It was a stupid question, irrelevant to the circumstances. "She's my daughter." I closed the door on them like they were intruders, allowing Anna and I to take what relief we could by being together. We had never been as close as we were in those first moments. Anna had been an enigma since high school, only allowing Don and me to see glimpses of her inner thoughts, never showing any weakness to mire her outward appearance of self-control. But now we were the same person, comingling our outpouring of pain, oblivious to anyone who might be observing.

As I sat on the couch hugging Anna, it seemed that I drew back and looked down on the scene from a distance. This shouldn't be happening. It was all a mistake. Don's depression was brought on by a drug. He didn't mean to kill himself. Why didn't I follow him when he drove off and explain this to him?

It had taken nearly five hours for the police to locate Don at Whale Rock Reservoir. I'd figured out where he had gone to take his life. My first thought was that he didn't have to die. It was a terrible mistake. Why didn't he understand that he took a drug and it made him bipolar, and then he got depressed and developed suicidal ideation? He wasn't really mentally ill. This is how I would explain Don's death to everyone the following days. I had to make them understand that it was an accident. I had to defend Don's honor. This wasn't supposed to happen.

All the while Don was planning to kill himself, I was convinced that things were improving and that they could only get better. While I was misinterpreting depression for a return to normalcy, Don was succumbing to the distorted messages from his brain. This is what I discovered too late in the search history on Don's computer:

> A firearm is not suitable for a suicidal gesture, as the chances of success are much higher than other methods.
>
> Possible effects of failing: Disfigurement, paralysis, pain, infection, brain damage, damage to liver, spleen, diaphragm, and collapsed lungs ("Firearms" 2018).

I didn't know then about the excitement the suicidal person can feel in planning his death. The process of finding the right place. The right method. The precision in the details. I realize now that he had bought the shotgun shells at Big 5 Sporting Goods. I found the receipt was in his drawer with the extra shells.

When I could finally talk, I called Don's brother Joe. He came over to make the calls to Don's other brother, Dave, in Ohio, and his sisters, Mary and Teri, who also lived in California. I couldn't sleep, so I stayed up with Joe and recounted the day's events over and over. I waited until the morning to call my son, John. He was in law school and had a class that day. I worried about what this would mean for him. He had a month to go before finals. I caught him right before his class. I think the words came out in a jumble, and I don't remember the sequence or details. John said I sounded detached.

"I'm sorry sweetie, but Dad is dead." I hurried on in the moments of silence, anxious to get it all out. "He shot himself with Grandpa's shotgun. He took off in the morning and he was gone all day. I didn't call the police until five because it took me awhile to realize he had the gun until after the movie. And I just kept hoping…" I didn't know the most important events to relate; they were all jumbled together.

John broke in crying. "I'll have to call you back, Mom. I'm standing in the parking lot by my classroom and I want to drive back home."

"I'm sorry. I tried to get you before you left for class." He had to absorb the news that his father was dead, and I still had to tell him that his father had planned it. Don had abandoned us.

There was someone else I had to talk to before I called anyone else.

"How could you have not known this?" I said to Dr. Lin when I contacted her later that morning. "It took me fifteen minutes on the internet to find this information about prednisone causing suicidal thoughts and the importance of monitoring. And it's from reliable sources." I cited publications and websites.

"You saw the way he was," I said. "You even said that if you didn't know him, you'd think he was scary." I kept driving for an answer I knew I wouldn't get. "That's when I asked you to please put him on something. Why didn't you listen?"

"What do you want from me?" Her voice finally broke from the professional tone she usually used. I'd gotten to her.

"Don't let this happen to anyone else."

"We have a psychiatrist now," she said, "to help us with patients like Don."

* * *

The treeless hills surrounding Whale Rock Reservoir were covered in a California drought-brown blanket of dead grasses romanticized by John Steinbeck as "fields of gold." Empty beer bottles and condoms lay in the weeds. Even a pair of men's faded blue Jockey shorts. I'd come seeking a meditative atmosphere; instead I was repelled by this juxtaposition of sex and death, but I still searched. The air was still, and plastic bags sagged in the star thistle like deflated lungs.

Why didn't I come here when I first suspected that Don might be suicidal, and this was the place he might be? I might have intercepted him, and I might have talked him out of it. Was it a lack of courage?

Reliving those moments, I see that I was afraid of what I'd encounter finding him dead or alive. What he might do to me and what I might see. The police showed me where they found him after they had cleaned it all up. And there's a lot to clean up after someone puts a shotgun in his mouth and pulls the trigger. They showed me the rock where Don could stay partially hidden from the road by lying at its base and using it to prop up his head and shoulders to position the shotgun correctly.

Where was the blood? Like the antithesis of Lady Macbeth in her vain attempts to wash away all the bloody guilt, I wanted to revel in it. But there wasn't a red stain on the granite rock or a dark area on the ground. The police report had said Don's body was found with "a large predominantly right skull defect with multiple skull fractures and avulsion of much of the cerebral cortex." This meant he had literally blown his brains out. For some reason it made me feel better to say it that way, to meet it head on. I knew the words shocked, but I found comfort in letting others know the true impact of what Don had done to himself. I enjoyed seeing expressions of horror when someone asked if I had to identify Don's body and I replied, "There wasn't much of his head left to identify." I knew this already because I'd read that:

> For those that discover the body of someone attempting a firearm suicide, the vision may well be traumatic. A shot to the head that has an exit hole is likely to spread blood and brain/bone fragments over a wide space. Depending on where the gun is aimed, it is also possible that bloody facial disfigurement occurs. A bullet not exiting the head will result in blood coming out of the entry hole ("Firearms" 2018).

I dropped to my knees in the prickly weeds and sifted through the dirt, looking for bone fragments like an archaeologist searching for remnants of a lost civilization. All I found were cigarette butts. I had expected a feeling of closure at finding Don's final resting place. Instead I was morbidly curious about why there would be no blood. What had they used to clean it up so thoroughly? Why hadn't they left some of him for me?

I sat by the rock and leaned back trying to see what Don would have seen. Normally I would have had a clear view of the ocean a good five miles away, but a layer of fog obscured the coast and snuggled against the cliff, moving swiftly toward me like a wave, sealing off any glimpses of life.

* * *

Don's memorial service seemed like a party. A friend had donated her beach house in Cayucos for the occasion and other friends had spread the word. Many of Don's former teaching colleagues were there, as well as neighbors and tennis buddies. Several cousins came up from Los Angeles. Death brings people together, makes them want to get back in touch. The crowd swelled and spilled out of the small backyard into the road. The ocean glistened in the background just across the street and beyond a few yards of sandy beach.

I didn't know many of the people there, and I hung with my family members. I was one of many celebrating Don's life.

I was happy to be left alone, not to have to listen to condolences anymore. The word *suicide* was difficult to avoid in such conversations, as were the euphemisms of how Don could "take his life," "kill himself," or "do something like that." The worst expression was, "at least he's at peace." I always had to argue back that Don was on prednisone and it made him do it. There's no peace in such a death for someone forced to kill themselves. "No," I usually said. "I feel as if Don has been murdered."

My brother-in-law Joe invited various friends and relations to speak about Don. The force of his personality was palpable, but I felt more like an observer. It was good to have Don honored that way; no religious observations were necessary to move people. The stories were mostly humorous, showing Don's strong nature, individualism, and enthusiasm.

Joe told a story about Don snorkeling with him in Hawaii, luring him out farther than he really wanted to go by taking a zigzagging route and pointing out different species of fish along the way. Joe was so distracted by the sights underwater he stopped worrying about how far out Don had led him. It wasn't until they returned to shore that Joe realized how far out he'd gone, way beyond the surf line. Don laughed and said, "You wouldn't have seen all of the different fish just by hanging out close to shore. Now you'll have a story to tell your grandkids."

Don's sister Teri told a story of how Don, as the oldest of six children, had gotten into some candy that was off-limits for the kids. When their parents found out, no one admitted to it. They were left alone in a room until the culprit confessed. Don looked at his younger siblings seriously, "We have a problem, and no one is going to admit they took the candy, right? And we all want to get out of here, right? So we can watch *Gunsmoke* on TV. I have a solution." Don then tried to convince his four-year-old sister, Mary, to take the blame because, as the youngest, she wouldn't get in so much trouble. Mary agreed to take the blame, but her parents didn't believe her because she wasn't tall enough to reach the candy jar. The expression on Don's face when he realized his plan had backfired did him in.

There were tennis stories recounting Don's prowess on the court and his irritation with his partners if they didn't do well enough. Of course, someone mentioned Don playing tennis with a cane when he was coming back from an injury. How he hobbled around the court batting back balls, still managing to make decent shots.

Dave Buck-Moyer, one of Don's friends who had taught middle school with him, had a story that drew knowing laughs from the crowd.

"One year, at the beginning of the school year, the superintendent had packed our classrooms full to accommodate extra enrollments, but there weren't enough desks in the classrooms. The district kept promising to reduce the numbers by hiring more teachers, but weeks went by with no changes. We all got together to draft a letter to the parents of our students with comments about the loss of quality instruction with fifty students in a class, and included photographs of students sitting on the floor, hanging out the windows, and trying to step over each other. Don volunteered to take the letter to our principal and superintendent and tell them that it would go out to the parents if changes were not made by the end of the week. Well, there was a lot of shuffling on that went on behind the scenes, but by Monday our class sizes were down to thirty."

John read a eulogy for his father:

> Thank you all for coming today to celebrate Don's life. Most of us know him as some combination of a family member,

teacher, coworker, mentor, and friend. As his son, I was lucky enough to love him as all of these.

Dad was always a fierce advocate for his family and friends. His loyalty meant unwavering support and help when you needed it most.

When I had trouble learning algebra, Dad sat with me at the kitchen table, and despite my best efforts, made what seemed like hieroglyphics into something I understood. His enthusiasm was infectious when he described what he was planning to do in his social studies classes and I saw that same enthusiasm in the faces of his former students when we came across them.

Anna and I spent many summers helping Dad take care of our house and property—cutting firewood, weed-whacking, and painting. Dad always made the effort to tell us how much he appreciated our help. I fondly remember relaxing with him after a hard day's work with a plate of carne asada tacos or a frosted mug of root beer and seeing his contented smile.

I turned to Dad for guidance throughout my life because he had a talent for making a bad situation seem manageable. When I talked to him about something troubling me, he listened carefully, asked thoughtful questions, and shared his thoughts in a way that showed his support, leaving me feeling empowered and ready to tackle the problem head-on. He was also a master of the strategically placed joke and bears much of the responsibility for my corny sense of humor.

Dad led me on some of my favorite adventures. We earned scars together mountain biking down ski slopes in the summer and clambering over the boulders on top of Bishop Peak. He taught me the value of seeking out new experiences, including a snorkeling trip where he encouraged me to follow him to see a "dogfish," which turned out to be a white tip reef shark hovering at the sandy bottom of a lava tube. As I fought the urge to frantically paddle away, I

> watched Dad dive down to the rim of the tube for a closer look. He taught me that sometimes you have to push your limits to live life to its fullest.
>
> When Dad was diagnosed with myelodysplasia, he found out that the average lifespan of people with his form of the disease was only two years. He managed the disease for over four and a half years with occasional treatments to boost his production of blood cells. He coped with a bone marrow transplant and the multiple complications that followed. He returned to the tennis court with a racket in one hand and a cane in the other. Even losing an ear to skin cancer did not dampen his resolve, and Anna referred to him as a "one-eared rogue." Dad had eleven years after that initial diagnosis and I am thankful beyond words to the people who helped him. I miss him every day, but I know the best way to keep Dad in my heart is to live the way he did: with compassion, empathy, tenacity, courage, and curiosity. I think that as long as we honor him that way, he will never truly be gone.

I found Don's memoir that night and started reading it to better see the man he was in his own words. As I picked through it I looked for any clues that might lead to a suicidal personality, but I found nothing from even the earliest time which would lead someone to believe Don could end up leaving this world in such a way.

It read:

> By fifty, I had unthinkingly fulfilled a prediction I'd heard in a graduate school class. The professor had said that his research had indicated that our society was in flux and that most college graduates would eventually change occupation five to seven times in their lifetimes. His prediction sounded ridiculous at the time. Nonetheless, it proved true for me. I'd been a probation officer, a school psychologist, a special education teacher, a math and history teacher, and a school counselor. I'd had five occupations by age fifty. During that time, I had been following the early strategy learned while my father tried so hard to help me learn to read. I'd tried to present a picture of the "perfect guy." I pictured what others would ideally like to see. I then presented them with that

persona. I defined myself in their vision of me. I tried to be the model school psychologist, counselor, teacher, etc. I'd been a chameleon blending into background of the role of the occupation.

On my fiftieth birthday, I told my family and friends that I'd decided to put a new self-motto into effect. I declared that I was going to "take no shit and take no prisoners" This was, of course, an exaggeration. I was serious about how I was going to approach the rest of my life. Until that time, the chameleon part of me had hidden some of my true personality. I'd hidden the intensity of various forces driving me. I'd hidden much of my competitiveness, my drive to excel, my need for recognition of my abilities and experience, my resentments about working with supervisors whom I thought inferior. I'd hidden the exhaustion of my patience after thirty years of appearing excessively calm and patient in the face of frustrating situations. I had realized that I'd created a storehouse of emotional internal baggage. I was unwilling to continue to add to the storehouse. I wanted to get rid of as much of this unnecessary emotional weight as I could.

My dad was a wonderful guy is many, many ways, but he was a fearsome force when angered. He would not back down or relent if he thought he was in the right. He was a model of indomitable will. I watched and learned; I internalized these lessons and kept them hidden. These early lessons would not overtly show until I had declared the "take no shit, take no prisoners" philosophy. This was in extreme contrast to the charitable, innocent altar boy, the "perfect child" role I had practiced for so long.

* * *

Don's service was the last time I saw many of his former friends and distant relatives. I realized that Don was a man who touched many lives and that he would be remembered. So often the person who commits suicide leaves behind fractured relationships and burned-out friendships. The decline is a progressively downward spiral until it is difficult to remember the person in any other capacity. But that wasn't true about Don.

I girded myself for the times to come when the comfort of friends and strangers would not be enough to fight my inner demons. Guilt has a way of presenting itself in strange ways. I had basked in Don's shadow since I met him, covering up my own insecurities. Before I met Don, I'd never had a serious relationship. I didn't plan on marrying until I was well established in a career. I was still running from an embattled family; my parents had divorced when I was nineteen. Don came into my life, I projected my emotional baggage onto him, and he took it all. He was interested in my problems and he wanted to help me.

Grief and its many manifestations made me look more closely at myself. I didn't know where Don's influence on me started and where I began—and where I was headed. My own deal with the devil was on the horizon.

Chapter 6
The Facade

After the family members left and went back to their postponed lives, Anna and I were left together to make our way through the challenges that lay ahead, sometimes dependent on each other. The initial bond we had felt when we first heard "I'm so sorry" from the police officers had gradually faded as conflicting emotions took over.

Anna had been living at home during Don's troubling time on prednisone, and she'd witnessed the utter deconstruction of her father's personality. In the wake of Don's passing, I assumed we'd recount those times and try to make sense of what had happened. But I didn't understand her needs, and she reacted to Don's death differently.

Anna cried a lot during the first days. I tried to comfort her by repeating, "He didn't mean to do it. We can get through this." We slept in the same bed because it was easier to fall asleep with someone there. I needed this more than Anna and I was sad when she returned to her own bed. I saw everything as a rejection.

At some point our emotional reactions diverged, and Anna took charge of the household, peering into the refrigerator and proclaiming, "This yogurt went bad, Mom. You should have eaten it up before you opened the new container," and making grocery lists while I read the paper and went for long walks. She became alternately annoyed and sympathetic. I tried to tread carefully around her, never knowing if I was friend or foe. I realized one night at dinner how different our perspectives were about Don's death. Often I'd muse about various aspects of the suicide, using Anna as my sounding board. I didn't realize how differently Anna saw things.

"I just can't believe it took the police so long to find Dad. I talked to the officer at five, and they didn't get out to Whale Rock until nine?"

Anna glared at me. "You've already brought this up a million times. You act like it was someone else's responsibility to find Dad and rescue him when he was probably already dead when you called the police."

"We don't know that," I said. "There were only vague references to the time of death, that rigor mortis had set in when they found him at ten o'clock."

"Mom, all these details don't matter. What I don't understand is why he didn't tell someone himself when he knew how bad it was. He had a background in psychology and counseling. He would have known to at least call a suicide hotline."

"He couldn't help it. When your brain is that distorted, you don't have any more control. You should read about this. I have all this information."

"I was a biopsychology major, Mom. I took neuroanatomy. I know about chemical influences on the brain. I'm saying that on some level he had control."

"He told me a few days before that he was afraid of his feelings. So, he did try to reach out. Maybe it's my fault he didn't get help in time. I waited too long." I hadn't wanted to reveal this, but I was willing to implicate myself to change Anna's impression of her father. "He'd never willingly abandon you."

"This isn't something I can talk about right now," she said. "I'm going down to meet some friends at the beach."

"We can talk later?"

"I don't know."

"I think you need to talk to someone. If you don't want to talk to me, will you talk to a psychologist?"

Anna paused by my chair. She smelled faintly of her lavender soap. Her eyes were tearful, but her voice was steady and strong. "Right now I don't want to talk to a psychologist because I'll probably start crying, and I'm tired of crying. I just want to go out and have fun with my friends and pretend that I'm normal."

Since adolescence Anna had kept her emotions to herself, rarely sharing personal problems or asking for advice. I left her alone, and I tried to be available to talk. Our personal dynamics weren't going to change in an instant.

We retreated into our own worlds. She drank to fall asleep. I took Don's leftover Ambien. Neither of us slept very well. I allowed us to whirl apart because I couldn't bear her rejection. I ignored the empty wine bottles as long as I never saw her drunk. And who was I to give advice?

I didn't reveal my anxiety to anyone. They would want me to do something. To take her somewhere. Not ignore her like I did Don. It was best to keep them away from any doubts they may have. Our recovery was going well, thank you, right according to schedule. She was resilient enough to make it. All I could do was watch and wait.

It has taken us time to understand how to be mother and daughter as well as friends. Anna knows that there is one person she can always count on for support when she needs it. I have learned the differences between our two perceptions of abandonment. For family survivors of suicide, the grief is complicated by abandonment. We both saw Don as a protector, but in Anna's case, the loss of her father at age twenty-three slammed shut a door in her life.

As for me, I had no control over my emotions, and trying to construct a rational explanation did not help. No matter how many times I heard, "It's not your fault," I thought I could have done more. I knew the doctors were responsible for not doing anything to help, but why didn't I go out to Whale Rock Reservoir myself? Don would have done it for me if our roles were reversed and he thought I would harm myself. I hadn't been there for him.

Even among people I felt alone, as if observing myself in this new state. I didn't relate to anyone, even other widows. In the wine section of the grocery store, I ran into a fellow teacher who had lost her husband to a heart attack a few years ago.

"I know what you're going through," she said. "Welcome to the club."

I wanted to take the time to explain to her while she picked out the best-priced Cabernet that a natural death is not like a suicide so, no, we were not experiencing the same thing at all. There were some hard questions I wanted to ask her: Could you have literally saved your husband's life? Do you know how it feels to replay events up to the last moments of your husband's life, digging for clues and warnings that you blame yourself for, not noticing or taking seriously enough? Do you know how it feels to tell your husband to "Die and go to hell," and ruminate on how, two months later, he shoots himself? Do you know how it feels to wake up every night in panic, not knowing what you fear? Can you say to me that you know what it feels like to realize that the person you once were has vanished?

I longed to disappear somewhere to a remote place and be taken care of. I didn't feel like I could function on my own, and I became highly anxious. I was afraid of driving. I wouldn't go on the freeway if I could possibly avoid it, and if I had to I'd creep along behind the trucks, driving as slowly as they did to avoid having to pass.

Perhaps, because of the anxiety, I could be overly aggressive. I found it infuriating when two construction workers parked their trailer on my property overnight when they were building a house across the street. I could see the ugly steel hulk from my kitchen window. The next morning, I spied them arriving at the site. I slipped on my bathrobe and UGG boots over my pajamas and ran out the door to intercept them before they drifted off.

"Hey! Hey you!"

They stopped and regarded me indifferently. This infuriated me more.

"Get your trailer off my property."

One of the men looked across the street to where I pointed. "That's your property?"

"Yes, it is. And I don't want any of your vehicles parked there."

"Since you asked so nicely, I guess we will move the trailer from your property."

"And since when did you ask me so nicely if you could park it there in the first place?"

I slogged back to my house indignantly; my UGGs scuffing up asphalt and my bathrobe flapping.

The gym became my refuge. It was close to my house, which meant I didn't have to get on the freeway. I spent hours a day on the cross trainer, the elliptical, the stair-stepper, the stationary bike. I wanted to get in control of my body again. I rotated on each aerobic machine sweating pools on the floor until I got the endorphin rush that passed for a moment's respite.

When I needed more to hold back the tidal wave of terror, I entered the weight room, normally a rather intimidating area of the gym, the domain of men and aggression. Alive with grunting and clanging and the loud thud of barbells dropped on the floor, it looked engaging, like it would help me control my body again. At least it would distract me from having to think and constantly question myself.

I saw a middle-aged woman who was struggling through some of the lighter equipment. Her name was Leila and she showed me how to adjust the seat for the pectoral fly and helped me lug a twenty-five-pound plate.

She took the bench next to mine and I spotted her for three sets of forty-five pounds. We were surrounded by grunting men. "Lordy, it's nice to have some female company in here," Leila said.

I had an hour of respite that day. I could concentrate on my muscle groups. Cycling and walking left too much brain-space for thinking. I returned the next day and worked on a different set of muscles. I watched someone using the free weights and copied some of the exercises they did.

Still giddy after my workout, I backed my car slowly out of the parking space, careful, as always, of other drivers. Look to the right, to the left. Then reverse. What? A car had stopped behind me. The door opened, and hairy legs appeared in my rearview mirror. Now a man was at my door, his face contorted under tangled hair. He was raging at me about me hitting his car. This car had come out of nowhere. He must have been driving too fast through the parking lot and not seen me slowly backing up.

Without thinking I launched out of my car and confronted the man, my hair wild after my workout. My rage came from a primal source wholly inappropriate to the circumstances but felt justified to me. He said he was in the "right of way." He pointed to a dent in the driver's side of his car door.

I screamed back, "You don't know what you're talking about." We argued about whose fault it was. In a second, I'd gone from a calm state to this off-the-charts explosion. He began to back down under the fury of my counterattack. I calmed down and we sullenly exchanged insurance information and a few last words about whose insurance was going to pay. I had to wait for a long time before my head stopped pounding and I felt like I could drive.

This was just one of many anxiety-inducing situations on the road. The details of the fender-bender incident kept reverberating throughout the week like shockwaves. Everything was grossly exaggerated, like I was in the *Car Crash* video game my son used to play. Cars I encountered driving up or down the hill to my house appeared to be headed directly toward me, veering off at the last moment.

I remember friends and family telling me how amazingly well I was doing. My sense of humor returned when I described my fender bender and "the hairy legs appearing in my rearview mirror." I didn't tell anyone about how anxious I had gotten.

They didn't know about me getting lost. They didn't know about all the clues I missed. I needed to talk things out. I needed someone to explain what was wrong with me, to tell me why I hadn't done more.

Chapter 7
Guilty as Charged

I went to Doctor Crosby ostensibly to ask about sleep and anxiety, but I kept bringing up guilt. She was in her late forties and petite, with an alluring self-confidence. Someone easy to talk to and easy to like. She wore a scarf loosely over her shoulders. I imagined her on weekends visiting the farmer's market wearing a straw hat and carrying a basket filled with fresh produce, carrot tops draping over the edge.

I sat across from her on a leather couch. I'd been here about fifteen minutes trying to get the courage to tell her about Whale Rock Reservoir. "I thought I knew where he was," I blurted out. "Why didn't I go there right away?" I said. "Maybe I could have talked him out of it?" I looked at her expecting answers.

She stared at me from across the room, the seating carefully arranged to discourage conversation and avoid intimacy. I looked at her books on the bookshelf. Among some psychiatry textbooks and a book about drugs, there was a collection of Anne Sexton's poetry. I liked the idea that she read poetry.

"One thing you have to know," she said, "this is not your fault. It was an impulsive decision."

"No," I said. "He planned it. I remember a few weeks before seeing something like a rifle in the backseat of the truck. I didn't think anything of it at the time. And I remember that he came home excited the day before he killed himself. He'd been at Whale Rock Reservoir, the place where he was found. When he was missing for so long, I thought he might have gone back there."

Dr. Crosby wrote something in her notebook. "From what you have told me, your husband should have been hospitalized when he became manic. He could have been observed there and given treatment. You are not responsible in any way for his death."

"But I told him to die and go to hell." I hadn't told anyone this yet. I was afraid of what they would think. That I would lose my heroic grieving widows status and their sympathy.

"People don't commit suicide because of what someone has said to them," she said. Now she leaned forward. "If he had told you to die and go to hell would you have done it?"

I shook my head, but the terrible cruelty of those words I'd said still haunted me. "I told him later I was really sorry. But I think that in some way I influenced him. I wanted so hard to hurt him, and I did. I could tell by the way he looked."

Dr. Crosby nodded in a noncommittal way to show she'd acknowledged what I'd said. "I think you will find support groups very helpful."

Support groups? More strangers? Sharing private stories?

"Don't you provide therapy? I know you, and I hoped you could see me."

"I wish I could do therapy, but I don't have time anymore."

"You don't do psychoanalysis?"

She laughed. "There's only one psychiatrist in town who still practices analysis."

She took a card from the table next to her chair. "Most of my clients in situations like yours find the best recovery from suicide survivor support groups and grief counseling. Hospice can help you with both."

I took the card from her and two prescriptions: one for Ativan for my sleeping problems and the other, Prozac, for my anxiety. As I left her office I passed her medical degrees hanging on the wall: Doctor of Medicine, Residency in Psychiatry. I'd had visions of lying on a couch getting questioned by Doctor Crosby with her chin in her hand asking pertinent questions about my dreams and anxieties.

I'd thought Doctor Crosby was going to flush out the demons.

* * *

My local hospice made it clear on its website that support groups were for suicide survivors, meaning: those family and friends who had known the person who committed suicide. Not to be confused with those who had "survived" a suicide attempt.

I got lost trying to find the address and stumbled onto a Christmas party. It was a warm evening and people wearing Santa hats were gathered on the front porch of a festively decorated house. Frank Sinatra was singing "Joy to the World."

I barged in on a circle of conversation. "Excuse me. Do any of you know where hospice is? I thought it was this address?"

"It's just down the street," someone said. "That big two-story on the corner. But if you can't find it come back and party with us."

The people on the porch looked like college students, and I wanted to join them, to go back in time to those days.

The hospice building looked like an unkempt halfway house. The gray paint and cracked steps gave off an unwelcome vibe, while cheerful sounds came from the direction of the party. Hospice probably didn't go for much glitter around the holidays. It was a time of depression for the mentally ill. I had to brace myself to enter. I understood why Anna had decided to go to a gathering with her friends.

Inside I found the meeting room and joined a circle of eight men and women. Instead of needles and yarn we held boxes of tissue. Everyone except me was crying, not the wailing of the first discovery, but the experienced tears of the anguish that follows. The quietness of the expression of grief was what impressed me. Our counselor, Mark, explained briefly that he was mostly going to observe, to remain in the background. It was our meeting. We were the leaders and ministers.

The first to begin was Madelyn, who had received a call from her brother while she was watching a movie. She didn't answer the call, but at the end of the movie, which was about the plight of killer whales kept in amusement parks, she began crying and had to remain in her seat while everyone else left the theater. "It was a sad movie, but not that sad. No one else was carrying on like me." Later, when she tried to call her brother back, he didn't answer. "I think he was calling to say goodbye and I missed his last words. Maybe I could have stopped him. Talked him out of it."

I wondered if I should tell her about Whale Rock Reservoir. How I sat for hours suspecting Don was there? That should make her feel better.

Cynthia was around fifty with a pixie face and short blonde hair. Through her tears she and her husband had adopted seven children and raised them on a ranch in Montana. She said both of her sons had committed suicide. The first one had PTSD from service in Iraq. The second son had shot himself only two years later. It was completely unexpected. "He called me in the morning on his way to work like he always did, and then he went somewhere and killed himself. I'll never know why." She looked down at her hands. "My husband and I thought that raising the kids on a ranch would be good for them. Let them work with their hands and get them away from all of the mischief of the cities."

Jennifer, who looked to be in her early twenties, began speaking. Recently married with no children of her own, she'd taken her sister's two young children away to escape a doomed world of heroin and abuse. Her sister had called to speak to her kids, and Jennifer had refused. "They just got so upset when she called. They'd cry for hours. And she'd only call when she came down. Then we wouldn't hear from her for weeks."

Her sister had overdosed the next day. Jennifer felt guilty because she hadn't allowed her sister the contact. Jennifer thought she contributed to the suicide somehow.

Something unearthly was happening in that room as we shared stories. We knew nothing about each other, yet we shared an experience no one else could understand. The atmosphere we had created was alive and authentic. There was no reason to hide any of the grief from each other. These people would understand my questions and my guilt. They had the power to forgive me because they knew what it was like to be in my place.

Here I could be soothed by the collective spirit like a meeting of druids in the forest but without the ghosts. It reminded me of a church I'd wandered into in the highlands of Chiapas. An old colonial cathedral that smelled of incense and pine. Indigenous women in blue cotton blouses and black woolen skirts knelt on the floor before small altars where they had placed offerings of food. They cried in the same quiet way, acknowledging that they were at another point in grief's cycle.

These people had gone through years of hell putting up with their family members and trying to support them, only to be left with the gift of guilt. I was getting angry, but not at Don. Don wasn't like these others. Don would never have done what these people did to their families. Some of them had made sure they took their families with them. Leaving a grieving mother like that a second time seemed to me like a distorted form of attention-seeking behavior. The addict who neglected her children did have choices to seek help. I thought of all the emotion that flows to the deceased. The attention that goes to the person who committed suicide when the real victims are the survivors. I didn't know what the protocol was, but I had to speak.

"You shouldn't feel bad," I said to Jennifer. "You saved those poor children. You're a heroine." I heard a few voices of support: "Who knows what would have happened to them if you hadn't interfered?"

Jennifer shook her head. "I stopped her from talking to them one last time. Maybe she wanted to say goodbye."

Lynn began speaking next. Her husband, Bob, sat mutely next to her with sad basset hound eyes. Their forty-year-old son, Aaron, had been an alcoholic for most of his adult life, spending years in and out of institutions. "But they wouldn't keep him," said Lynn, her voice quavering. Aaron had been living with Lynn and Bob as he battled another bout of depression when it happened. "We came home from shopping and found him." Her voice trailed off. "He knew where the gun was."

I was the only one left who hadn't shared my story. I was unsure of what to say. My anger burned too strong for what had happened to Don, and I felt compelled to point out how he was different. "I'm sorry for the loss of your loved ones," I said. "And I don't think my husband was any better than those you lost. But my husband wasn't a drug addict or an alcoholic nor did he suffer from bipolar disease—not really. He was just fine, and then he took a drug that made him psychotic. I begged his doctors to get him help, but they refused. They said he'd be fine if they just tapered him off the drug. The whole thing was a big mistake. He didn't want to kill himself. He was forced to do it."

No one seemed to know what to say to me. Then someone spoke. "At least he's at peace now."

I knew this was meant to help, but it was the wrong thing to say and showed how impossible it was for me to explain why I thought it was prednisone's fault—Don had been hijacked. "No, he's not at peace," I said. "He went somewhere, and he shot himself. He was driven to do it. He was taken over by something, redirected. It was not Don pulling that trigger. If he is in a state where he's aware of what he's done, how could he feel anything but horror knowing that he could have been helped through this? He wanted to live, and his prognosis was good. If he hadn't had access to that stupid gun, we might have had time to get him help."

I heard some murmurs of agreement from Cynthia, the woman who'd lost two sons, and Jennifer. But Aaron's mother Lynn, who had said "he knew where the gun was," shook her head. "He could have found another way."

"I don't know for sure what he might have done," I said. "But I did find a website he'd been on about how to commit suicide painlessly and most efficiently, and a gunshot wound to the head is the way to do it."

Mark, maybe sensing that we'd veered off topic, said that our session was over, and as we filed out the door the spell that had bonded us was broken. We became strangers again. Lynn and Bob lingered beside me, and I feared that they might want to continue the gun debate. "I'm glad you came," Lynn said. "I think the authorities let me down too. I begged them to institutionalize Aaron because I was so worried, but they'd only hold him for three days."

Lynn hadn't listened to what I'd said. Don's and Aaron's situations were entirely different. They only shared the fact that they'd committed suicide. I wanted this place to be my refuge, my church, but I would always feel like I had to keep explaining about Don, about why my situation was different. I felt compassion for the families, but as a remote observer. I had nothing more to share with them and decided not to return.

It took time for me to see that it wasn't just the difference between Don and the others that made my situation unique. Guilt was on the table, but I couldn't talk about my guilt—Whale Rock Reservoir and how I waited so long when I suspected Don was there. There is honorable guilt like the kind I'd heard expressed in the circle of survivors. But I felt that my guilt was different because I could have done something. I might have stopped Don or at least called someone to go out and stop him.

Chapter 8
Grief 101

That winter of 2014, I started living inside my head, not really connected to my day-to-day reality. Time passed incrementally. Going grocery shopping could take hours. My unshared guilt lay in my subconscious, ready to torment me in ways Freudian analysts would delight in. I needed someone to tell me why I didn't go to Whale Rock Reservoir. I had a recurring dream that began a few nights after Don died. We were lying in bed, and I'd feel his hands caressing my body, but I couldn't see his face. I'd feel strong desire for him, pulling him toward me. When he rose above my body it wouldn't be his face I saw, but a grinning joker's face mocking me, lips pulled back in a lascivious leer, laughing when I squirmed and kicked to escape it. A demon had taken Don's place in my bed. This was what I deserved. This demon would pull out all the stops, had all the personal data of my life packed away to taunt me forever.

Other times I would revisit scenes from the past when I should have shown strength of character and determination but felt I hadn't. These occurred most frequently at night. One day I drove by a high school and remembered a time thirty-five years ago when I'd been helpless in the face of a gang attack.

It was my first year of teaching. I was assigned English and drama at Lincoln High School in southeast San Diego, known for its high drop-out rate, violence, and gangs. Having come of age in sixties and seventies when teaching was considered a noble profession, Don and I felt inspired to make a change in society: Don, by teaching students with learning disabilities, and me, by teaching high school to what were referred to as "underprivileged" high school students.

I'd talked to other teachers at the school and been given advice about motivating my students, many of whom had poor reading abilities and discipline issues. Being tough from the first day of class was the most often repeated advice, which was not my forte. I mistakenly thought that if I was just nice and positive, they would all respond in kind.

Though I usually got along well with my high school students, sometimes one would come along who needed a firm hand, and I wouldn't be able to do what was necessary like other teachers did with their force of personality. Rather than send them to Mr. Cook, the vice principal in charge of discipline, I'd keep them after class and try to wheedle them into being good.

One such student was Alan, who scared the hell out of me. There was a highly menacing quality about him. He'd look down at his desk most days, checked out, rarely participating in class and hardly ever completing assignments. When I spoke to him specifically, he'd look up with eyes narrowed, giving me the most hostile look, and grunt, "Huh? Leave me alone if you know what's good for you."

Taken aback by the look and being a new teacher in a different environment, I let it pass even though I should have reported him to Mr. Cook. I thought he'd warm up to me if I gave him a break. He saw through me. The nicer I was, the more he scowled. I also knew that Alan had a criminal background and had served time in juvenile hall.

One day I took a chance. The class had an assignment to write a poem. I called on Alan to read his after I saw him extract a folded-up piece of paper from his pocket. He never did homework assignments.

He smoothed the paper down and started reading. "Every day I come to school. / I have this English teacher who thinks she's cool, / but everyone knows she's just a fool."

"OK, Alan," I interrupted. "That's enough." The rest of the class was quiet, all eyes on me. My face was hot. I had to do something. "Alan, I think you better go down and show that to the vice principal."

He glared at me. "You kicking me out for doing my homework?"

"You know why I'm asking you to leave," I said. "What you wrote is very disrespectful."

"No, no," he said slowly. "Can't do that. Cook said I'd get suspended if I got kicked out of class one more time."

I was stuck between needing to stand up to him yet not knowing what to do if I continued to pressure him. If he felt backed into a corner, what might he do? I decided to back down and report his behavior when class was over. "Then stay after class so we can discuss this." I then went on with the lesson. Alan balled the paper up and threw it across the room at me. Then he stalked out of the classroom.

After I reported him to the vice principal, Alan didn't return to my class. But one day, in the middle of a literature assignment about the Harlem Renaissance, four tough-looking young men appeared at the doorway. They looked too old to be students, and they wore the blue bandannas of one of the local gangs. At first I ignored them, hoping they were just passing through the building on their way somewhere and had stopped by my room out of curiosity. Soon they'd get bored and leave before the security guard made his rounds.

"White bitch," they shouted. "We're going to get you."

I was afraid they'd come into the classroom. I was on the third floor of the building, on the end. They apparently came up an outside stairway and snuck past the security guards. I could have called out down the hallway for help or canceled class, hoping to keep the students safe. Instead, I continued to read. The gangbangers lurked outside the doorway, continuing with "white bitch."

Then the students took over. Growing up in the area had given them skills at handling situations that scared me. Two of my students, Jason and Michael, went out into the hallway with the men. They spoke quietly a few moments gesturing, looking back at me, shaking their heads, and then came back in grim-faced. "I still say we should jack her car at least," the men said, still standing at the door. But eventually they left.

The students told me that Alan had gotten suspended because of the previous incident in my classroom and had been sent to juvenile hall again for getting into trouble. He'd sent his friends to get me, saying I was a racist.

"Mrs. Stegman, they would have hurt you if we hadn't gone out there," Michael said. "We told them you were really cool."

I went to see Mr. Cook later that day to tell him about the confrontation. "I thought these guys were really going to hurt me," I said, in a quavering voice.

Payton Cook was a powerfully built African American man who took no bullshit from anyone except the superintendent. He had promised to clean up the school and make it a safe place for students and staff. He always had a frown on his face, even when he occasionally joked at staff meetings as if we weren't supposed to laugh. When he walked the halls several times a day, students ran away, not wanting "the stare" to land on them.

I felt meek sitting in his office relaying the details. The incident would have been a mere hiccup in his day.

"You should never have let this get so out of hand," he said when I told him about Alan's continued disrespect. "If the press gets ahold of this story, it's going to look bad for Lincoln High, and you know they're always looking for bad things to report." It was during a time when violence in the schools was a popular topic in the media. It seemed like every day there was an account about a stabbing or shooting at a school. "It will look like I'm not taking care of things." He tapped a pencil on his desk.

I felt like a piss ant sitting before him. I was a pale 120-pound lightweight. His bulky shoulders looked like they'd pop the seams of his suit jacket, and his face was usually set in a scowl. My discipline problems would vanish if I looked like him. "I'll try to do better," I said. "But I don't know how I could have stopped those guys. They came right in off the street."

Cook gave me an appraising gaze. "I can see you're really scared," he said. "And that makes me wonder if you're right for Lincoln High."

"I do want to be here," I said plaintively. As a first-year teacher it was his call as to whether I'd be back. Being fired from this job would have been the end of my teaching career.

"Well then you need to toughen up to teach here."

I stayed out of Cook's way for the rest of the year and even put on a play, which hadn't been done in ten years. Mr. Cook beamed from the audience on opening night. Fortunately, I never had another student like Alan to confront, but I transferred from the school before I could have the chance to challenge myself again.

Sitting in my car thirty-five years later, I relived the event as if it had just happened. It was one of many times I'd be reminded of something that happened years ago as proof of my lack of character. It was brutal self-analysis. Time after time it seemed that I did nothing when I should have shouted for attention. The same way I'd been with Don's doctors or those hours I'd waited, knowing where Don was.

I hadn't counted on such a powerful foe in the face of such situations: fear. It had paralyzed me then and was having the same effect on me years later. I would later learn that fear isn't always bad. It can be a warning signal and protection for fears known and unknown. Sometimes you must face confrontations and sometimes you run.

* * *

I was floating on what I could salvage of my life, endless days bobbing in a sea of routine answers to "How are you doing?" Sometimes I told people what I thought: "I feel like Don's been murdered," and watch them back away. Sometimes I gave a feel-good serene reply where I sounded falsely spiritual: "It's hard but I'm coping. Others have lost their spouses and managed. One dies and the other is left alone."

I thought I could make it through this way, just by going through the motions. But the nights alone were terrifying, and as darkness fell I was unable to escape the looming future, facing all the fears accumulated over time that manifested as aloneness. I didn't know who I was alone, and I had to reinvent myself. Was this grief?

Few understood how I felt. Some married friends, who had been alone for weeks when their husbands had traveled, said they enjoyed the time to themselves, relishing moving through the day solo unencumbered by the expectations of a cemented relationship. The haunting void of years ahead alone appeared like a black hole into which spun the fragments of my life.

The Ativan stopped working and my nights became a series of light sleeping punctuated with abruptly waking in a heightened state of anxiety, my mind seeming to work against me, remembering fragments of past bad behavior: cursing at my sister-in-law, spanking my daughter over spilled milk, refusing to accept my dying mother-in-law into our home during her final weeks of life.

Dr. Crosby told me I'd have to taper off of it I since my body had grown dependent.

"You mean I'm addicted to it?"

"We don't use that term for this. Tapering is similar to withdrawal, but not nearly as severe." She hesitated. "You'll be fine in a few weeks."

"What do I do now for sleeping?"

"You can try some natural sleep aids from the health food store. Some have found those beneficial." She had no particular brand to recommend. "Experiment with a few, and you might find something. Remember that grief counseling may help."

I'd been skeptical of natural sleep aids as unproven, faulty, and expensive alternatives to pharmaceuticals, but I tried every sleep aid I could find: valerian, magnesium, wild lettuce, and hops, but none could combat the thrust of anxiety that blasted through my sleep at regular intervals. I needed something to face the endless nights, so I chose vodka. It didn't help me sleep through the night, but it got me to sleep. I began drinking after dinner, welcoming the numbness through the evening, watching the bottle, which used to last months, disappear in a week.

Anna was alarmed one night to see me stagger down the hall. I thought I was fine until I stood up from the recliner, but I did feel dizzy. She retrieved one of the empty bottles from the trash. "I didn't know you were drinking so much of this. You just used to drink wine."

"I didn't drink it all. You drank it too. I saw you mixing it in your Sprite." Here I was, like an alcoholic in denial. I took the bottle to the sink and watched it chug down the drain.

"I didn't drink any of this. I stopped drinking months ago. I can tell you from personal experience, Mom. This isn't helping you."

Because everything else had failed, I decided to give the grief counselor a chance. I called hospice again and made an appointment. I wanted someone to tell me what was wrong with me and to talk to me instead of handing out pills. Jane Rankin was a woman in her forties with an empathetic smile. At our first meeting she sat directly across from me. "So, tell me what you are experiencing right now."

I launched into the familiar territory of summarizing the history of Don's mania on prednisone, my feeble attempts to get help from the doctors, their refusal, and Don's suicide. "He planned it. He blew his brains out. His death was a huge mistake."

She took notes the whole time and put her notebook away when I finished. "What I heard was an account of your husband's story delivered in an unemotional manner with numbness, not grief. Now that I know this background, let's hear Jill's story."

I was supposed to cry to convince her I'm grieving? "I don't know how to show emotion. I can just tell you what it is I'm feeling."

"Well, right now, the emotion I see and hear in you is anger. Lots of anger toward the doctors who could have intervened. But your grief must be addressed at some point for you to recover from this tragedy."

"What does grief look like? How do I know besides crying and sobbing and feeling sad?" I was growing weary of this grief business. "The anger feels real to me right now."

"Grief takes many forms, and anger can be part, but not all of it. You may be frightened of the process, and that's normal. Tell me, besides anger, what is bothering you the most?"

"I'm terrified of being alone."

"Why? What are you afraid of?"

I didn't know how to describe the haunting anxiety of being alone, the fear of becoming an eccentric bag lady or a negative personality reinforcing my own stereotypes and misconceptions.

"I'm afraid of myself and what comes to me at night when I'm alone. It all comes back."

Jane, as she had me call her, nodded for me to continue.

"What things come back?"

"All the things I could have done to help Don. How I could have driven out to Whale Rock Reservoir. How I could have intervened earlier. Why did I just sit there like a dumbass for so long?"

"So that's where the anger comes from? It's toward yourself, because of your guilt?"

"No, it's toward the doctors because they are the reason I'm feeling this way. The doctors and the medical establishment didn't help, and I wasn't aggressive enough to force them. It's not as if my husband is dead, la-de-dah, and now I'll cry and grieve and go through some predetermined process. It all comes back to the fact that Don shouldn't be dead. I can't separate out grief from the rest of it, and if I sound blunted and unemotional when I tell the story, it's because that's the way I deal with it."

Jane deflected my anger with a smile. "You definitely don't sound unemotional now. Anger is part of the process. It's just not good to be stuck there."

I was still unsure of what grief felt like, but I wanted to experience it so that I could move through the steps of recovery. I'd attempted to explain Don's death to anyone who would listen, but no one said anything that made me feel better. One friend told me she allowed herself an hour to grieve the death of her mother when the pain overwhelmed her. I remembered when my mother died, and I wished that I could process my grief that way, find the emotional link to its expression, allow myself to purge. If I could only understand what I was supposed to feel, I could "begin the process to recovery" that Jane Rankin described. But every time I looked in the mirror, I saw an alien, not a widow.

I was determined to be a good griever so that Jane could check me off and send me on my way. I wanted her approval that I was displaying grief because she might be right; a few tears could make me feel better. During our next few meetings, I sniffled a little and pretended to choke up, and Jane smiled approvingly at me, later writing in her notes: "Jill was a bit teary this time, breaking through the numbness."

I celebrated Jane's approval of my display of grief with another vodka-infused evening. Anna was away for the next five days, so I dragged the bottle out of its hiding place under bags of frozen vegetables. I tried to flee in sleep, but the joker appeared again in a dream wearing the same wicked grin, letting me know that I was not fooling myself.

I continued to find ways to impress Jane with my recovery by reading about the process of grief and trying to fake my way through the counseling sessions, even though it was counter to what I was truly feeling: I felt anger at what had happened to Don, not sadness. I saw Jane five more times. After the final visit Jane wrote: "Jill is doing well with her grief issues. She has decided to try dating and considers it a learning experience, but is concerned that it might be too soon. She was happy that I wasn't concerned. She would like to continue to establish new routines in this year following her husband's death."

I'd fooled my therapist, but I knew something was very wrong with me. My fear of being alone had grown to horror. I had depended on Don for emotional interaction since I'd run from the emotional insecurity of my family. Without him to reflect my emotions, I had no way of knowing who I was. I couldn't explain how it became a daily chore to face now every loss and mistake I'd ever made.

Chapter 9
Time Online

The joker-demon continued to appear in my dreams. He recalled a dormant part of my life I'd thought was probably extinct. I began sensing, unrealistically, that men I encountered had an interest in me. This idea was not based on any particular sign from them, but rather a perceived idea that I emitted a mysterious sexual pheromone, a talisman from the man I tried to escape in my dreams. I rummaged through the closet to find clothes that emphasized my curves. I wore turtlenecks to hide my sagging neck and sunglasses to cover the purplish bags under my eyes.

Our auto mechanic, fifteen years younger, had known both of us for over ten years. I'd broken down on the freeway, and he'd kindly stayed open until the tow truck arrived. I thought he looked at me differently when I paid the bill for the repairs. He seemed to be staring at me intently when I handed him the check. I wore knit pants that flattered me from the waist down. "Thank you so much for taking care of my car," I said. "You went above and beyond for me." I decided to be bold and leave an opening. "I'd like to repay you somehow. Would you like to come to dinner with my daughter and me?"

"That's nice of you," he laughed. "But it's not necessary. I really liked Don. He reminded me of my older brother who died a few years ago. It makes me feel good to keep his car running."

Not long after, I told my twin sister, Jean, about another dream where Don appeared at a party but was avoiding me. Standing right beside him, I tried desperately to get his attention, but he turned away to talk to someone else. The joker was there laughing at my vain attempts. Jean liked to apply her amateur psychology skills to dream interpretation. She'd studied Carl Jung and believed that dreams can be used to make decisions about her life. "It means it's time to move on," she said with her usual self-confidence. "You need more inputs in your life so that you won't be constantly inside your head."

Jean wasn't a psychologist, but her advice was based on her experiences, including a BA in psychology. She'd also studied "depth psychology" at a New Age college called Pacifica Institute. She decided that what I needed was distraction and a more active social life that would get me out of the house at night. She had discovered online dating and loved to show off the profiles of her admirers, a strange array of sixty- to seventy-year-old malcontents with histories of questionable relationships. One guy had been married and divorced three times to women many years younger. The last woman had been eighteen to his sixty. "I can overlook a lot," Jean said, "but I hold the line on smoking. I refuse to date a smoker." When that relationship took off, it fizzled after a month or so when the "boyfriend" told my sister to lose weight.

Jean was scrolling through men on her dating app. "Dwayne says I'm the most compatible woman he's ever been with," she said. At sixty-five, she'd been a widow for nearly twenty years, and she loved giving me advice. "He brought me flowers on the first date. How about that for a keeper?" She twisted the gold chain around her neck and crossed her legs. She wore new shorts, which showed off her calves and distracted from the folds of her mid-section. Her chin-length auburn hair was faded but showed no gray.

"Next week Dwayne's coming down in his BMW convertible and taking me to the Chumash Casino."

"But you don't even like gambling," I said. "And you said he smokes. That's two strikes."

"I know. I know. In a perfect world that's true. But this is a new era. Time to move on." She gave me a look. Don had been dead eighteen months. "Toleration is in. There are ten of us women to every man on these dating sites."

"What about ED?" I said, referring to what she'd informed me is rampant among men over sixty.

"That was the problem with those older guys," she said. "But Dwayne's forty-nine. I'm officially a cougar." She giggled. "He washed my car for me naked, and I took a video of it. Want to see?" Before I could say no, she scrolled on her cell phone and held it in front of my face.

Dwayne was leaning over her car displaying an erect penis in one hand, a garden hose in the other. I looked away. "What guy would do this on a date with a woman he hardly knows?"

"Naked dating is the new thing according to Ellen DeGeneres," my sister said. "Anyway, don't you think he's cute?"

"I think he's disturbed." I tried to imagine my sister cavorting about with Dwayne. It wasn't a stretch to imagine me in similar circumstances. The scene was decidedly not titillating. "This is really sick."

Jean put her phone back in her purse. "Well, I think you're the one who's disturbed. Are you still seeing the grief counselor?"

"I don't need grief counseling anymore," I snapped back. "I was signed off, told I'm fine now. A few sessions and, *voilà*, no more grief."

"I went through grief too," she said. Her voice broke. "So, I know what it is."

"You do know something about grief." I stopped myself from adding, but your husband died of a heart attack. And suicide trumps a heart attack.

"What about the psychiatrist?" she persisted.

"She just wanted to give me Prozac."

"There are other psychiatrists."

"That's what they all do now. There's a pill for everything." I saw where this line of questioning was going.

"You've turned into a humorless, scowling old woman and I'm just trying to help you have a little fun," she said. She picked up her purse and stalked out.

Jean was right about me, I felt dark compared to her liveliness and her enthusiastic embracing of new relationships. But our motivations were different. It wasn't the sex I missed, and it wasn't really companionship either. I'd been watching older couples. Leaning in close to catch snatches of conversation, all the mundane comments that made up a long-term relationship. Secretly examining every glance, every touch. Trying to guess how long they've been together.

The air around the couples was heavy and ripe. I missed what they had; the kinetic energy that formed stars could only happen between two poles. I was envious of the force-field around them, exuding their self-containment and wholeness. Alone, I was just an imploded planet, dead and sterile. People do lose their spouses and partners, and the world is full of we who are left behind, just as the universe is crowded with debris from shattered stars.

Soon I found myself browsing a "seniors" dating site, for those over fifty-five. I don't know how I got there. My hands seemed driven to the keyboard and my fingers forcibly pressed on the keys like my piano teacher did to me when I was seven. A hundred pictures of men in my area aged fifty to sixty-eight popped up: men by cars, men on boats, men straddling motorcycles, men holding fish. Fish? Were they looking for someone to clean them? So many men. By the fiftieth photo they all started looking the same: baseball caps to cover bald spots, Cheshire-cat grins, or expressionless, their features eclipsed by the sag of age. And the discovery that most were looking for younger women, sometimes ten years younger than me. By the time I eliminated all the sixty to sixty-five-year-olds not looking for a woman under forty-five, I'd winnowed the results down to ten who lived nearby. The dating site sent me a message that I might consider expanding my parameters. I decided I'd go up to sixty-nine, but not a year older.

While I browsed and mostly discarded the new selections of older men, the monitor began flashing. Someone named Marty from the dating site wanted to chat online. His photo showed a slim, sixtyish man with sensitive eyes. After a short exchange, I found out that he adored his two children and was expecting his first grandchild. That night he was making shrimp scampi for his pregnant daughter and her husband. After an hour I gave him my cell number.

My phone rang with an unfamiliar number and I answered it. Suddenly I was transformed from married to single and my throat tightened. I tried to sound natural, but I didn't sound like me. I reverted immediately to my childhood shyness. My parents had told me to bring people out by asking questions about themselves. I asked a question, Marty answered, and then I asked another. He mentioned he'd been married and divorced three times. I asked about his exes.

"My last wife was a mess. She got drunk at my daughter's wedding and made a scene."

"Where do you find these women?" I said.

"Everywhere," he laughed. "My brother says I just like to bring home stray cats."

Two hours later I was exhausted. My earlobe throbbed from the pressure of the phone. I knew everything about Marty and he knew nothing about me. Now he was talking about his depressed second ex-wife and how she killed herself. Seeing an in, I blurted out, "My husband committed suicide too. He shot himself."

In the silence that followed I was shaking. Why in the hell did I reveal that? Then Marty responded, "Oh my God. I'm so sorry," and soon said goodbye. Did I really expect to have a conversation about our mutual experiences with suicide? I couldn't believe the word still lurked in my subconscious, ready to assert itself like a bomb. I sat in the darkness feeling empty and more alone than ever. Outside my window, the crescent moon leered like the joker who followed me at night.

Maybe I expected a natural bond to occur? Many of the men said in their profile that they were looking for a spark. What spark? Physical attraction? I wasn't sexually attracted to Don when we first met; it was more of a friendship. But before him I had a romantic and naïve idea that I could trust anyone who wanted me. I mistook lust on their part for love. I took risks in pursuit of a fantasy romance.

When I was eighteen, I was nearly raped when I went home with a stranger I'd met on the street. It was 1968. I thought he just wanted to talk about politics. When he put his hands around my neck and forced me into his bedroom, I looked him in the eyes and asked about his mother. Would she be ashamed of what he was doing? He had me pinned to the wall, his mouth clamped shut, his jaw muscle twitching. I babbled on about a mother's love for her son while trying to maintain eye contact. He slowly released his grip on my throat, and I had to support myself so that I wouldn't crumple. I was lucky.

I trusted men too much, and I clearly didn't understand the sexual motives. My first year of college, I went down to San Diego with a friend, her boyfriend, and his friend. I didn't realize that I was supposed to hook-up with this strange man, at least that's what he had in mind. I did get in bed with him fully clothed, mostly because I was too drunk and sleepy to stand up any longer. He fell on the bed beside me and began fondling my breasts. I kicked at him and he rolled away. A few hours later he was at it again. This time he was on top of me. I felt his penis harden against my stomach. He was trying to pull my jeans down.

"Get off of me." I pushed against his chest, but he clamped me down harder. At some point he seemed to realize that he was forcing me against my will. That this wasn't what I wanted. He stopped pushing and grinding on me and I squirmed out from underneath him. I grabbed my purse and ran out of the motel room in the middle of the night.

"What a bitch," I heard him say behind me.

I didn't know what to do, but I wasn't going back in that motel. I saw what a mistake I'd made and how it must have looked to the guy. I couldn't face the scenario of driving back to UCLA with him and my friend and her boyfriend snuggling together in the backseat. I felt hurt and betrayed that someone would only think of me as a sex object. I was lucky again.

I knew Don as a friend then. We had gone out together but weren't yet romantically involved. I found him the easiest man to talk to. We spent hours walking on the beach discussing the art house movies of Federico Fellini and Ingmar Bergman. We went to see Miles Davis during his *Sketches of Spain* phase. We saw Jimi Hendrix play in a classroom at UCLA right before he became mainstream. We talked about religion—he was a Catholic then—and how it jived with the existentialist novels of Kafka, Vonnegut, and Hesse. Don was well read. His arguments were based on sound thinking and indisputable intelligence.

I located a phone booth, scraped together some change from my purse, and I called Don at his apartment in Manhattan Beach. I don't know why I called him and not one of my other friends. I just knew he'd help me.

He was puzzled that I'd gotten myself into such a situation. "You're in a motel in San Diego?" he said.

"No, I *was* in a motel, and now I'm on the street. I was with this guy, and I got drunk with him in a motel room, and I don't know what to do because he drove me down here." I sounded like a fool.

"Did he hurt you? Did he—?"

"No, he backed off finally when I yelled at him. I just can't face him anymore. You were the first person I thought of to call."

"I'm glad I was home. I just got off work." Don worked at the airport and usually had night shifts. "Do you want me to come down and get you?"

"Yes, please come and get me." It's what I wanted more than anything.

"OK, I'm coming, but it will take me a couple of hours. Are you in a safe place?"

"Yes," I said. "I'm at the Circle K on the corner of Ocean Boulevard and Nimitz."

When Don pulled up two hours later, I ran over and hugged him. He was still in his work shirt and he smelled like gas fumes. In his rush to get here, he hadn't even stopped to shower. His shirt felt soft and I rubbed my eyes on it to brush away my tears of relief. I noticed that his torso was a perfect V-shape from years of surfing and outdoor sports, which made me cling to him harder and in a sexual way. "Jills, Jills," he said. "I'm here now." I loved him then. He was a friend, brother, and lover all in one.

Don and I became inseparable after that. He listened to my other past dating experiences. "You need someone to look after you," he said when I told him about the near rape from before. I was nineteen and he was twenty-one.

I don't know what would have happened to me if I hadn't met Don. I was safe for the next thirty-five years. Then he was gone and I was transported back to the default mode of my youth: awkward shyness and hope that someone would come along who liked me.

I thought of those men I'd known before my husband and how they would be now, in their sixties. As young people we fit into categories. Names like college drop-out, druggie, greaser, hippie, surfer, thug, gangbanger, yuppie, nerd, and slut. You had to be something. I wondered how we would be categorized now, in late middle age, other than a former something? Aside from the men I knew from high school and the early days of college who were clearly headed for prison, did the others assume the roles society expected of them? The only "types" clearly identifiable to me in my age range were motorcycle misfits with Santa Claus beards and bellies to match and the occasional old hippie, with his ubiquitous gray ponytail, perpetually attired in flip-flops, drab T-shirt, and shorts. A full-bearded man in his sixties wearing a flannel shirt and too-short pants would not be labeled a hipster. He would more likely be described as seedy.

I had to prepare for these life changes. I realized that, aside from the men who chose to identify with a particular subgroup, most men my age looked the same, with similar clothing and hairstyles. Assumptions about how people looked at the world could not be taken for granted. A man with a ponytail could revere Ralph Nader or Rush Limbaugh. Would any of them want to take the time to understand me? Did I have the desire to take the time to know someone?

I knew that my loneliness made me vulnerable. I read that scammers were looking for widows and women in their sixties. Scammers fed on the high rejection rates of this group. My online dating accounts were filled with suspicious emails from men who always seemed to be traveling but were ready to "find true love and settle down."

After I mixed myself my cocktail of the week—a recipe concocted by my friend, consisting of two shots of vodka, a shot of Grand Marnier, two tablespoons of lemon juice, and a tablespoon of mint—I was back online again later that night, drawn to the photos of men on motorcycles, dazzled by the black-leathered forms astride their gleaming chrome machines. One guy had multicolored tattoos squiggling down his arms to his wrists. The lines intertwined down his muscular biceps and thick forearms like mating boa constrictors. His features were obscured by a black helmet. His written profile was short and barely intelligible:

"Hey u and me get 2 see how it works. I like to touch. Here's my number." He was making some kind of sign with his fingers. It could be a gang sign. Maybe something else. I liked the coarse communication, the poetry of its primitive call. I could reinvent myself, be someone new. I imagined myself with this faceless man on the back of his motorcycle challenging the wind, my arms around his waist, molded to his back with my fists squeezing tightly into his belly. My instincts were better now. I knew they were. I dialed the number.

Zack was the name of my motorcycle man. I met him in a safe area of the city park, beside the *Wood Nymphs*, a three-tiered fountain topped with three naked women cast in marble, which I thought would make a classy meeting place before I was whisked away on a black stallion/motorcycle. I'd always received compliments about my youthful appearance, but recently no one had recoiled in amazement when I told them my age.

When I spotted a frail-looking man sitting on a bench by the fountain, I couldn't believe it was the same sturdy-looking guy from the dating site. I considered veering off in another direction, but he stood and waved, "Are you Jill?" I saw that indeed he was very thin and sickly, and I realized his profile photo was not a recent one.

"I guess you're Zack?" He lightly grasped my hand in an anemic handshake. "How are you?" I couldn't determine what he thought about me because his eyes only seemed to register physical pain. I could see he weighed less than I did, and I weighed 140.

"I can't talk for long because of this pain in my jaw." He held his hand to his jaw and mumbled like his mouth was numb from a recent visit to the dentist. "I didn't want to tell you on the phone about it 'cause you might not have wanted to meet me. The doctor said there might be a tumor growing in there."

"I can't believe you're interested in meeting people if you don't feel well."

He smiled sadly. "Yeah, I haven't been able to eat anything but protein shakes for a few months because of this, so I guess going out to a restaurant isn't something I can do right now."

This meeting was far from what I'd expected. How could he possibly be looking for a girlfriend? What he needed was a nurse, and I wasn't going to fill that role even if I felt sorry for him. I asked him questions about doctor's visits, possible treatments, and other medical questions as if we had been two strangers striking up a conversation in the waiting room of a doctor's office. It was familiar territory for me having been to so many appointments with Don.

"You seem to know lots about medical stuff. I would have thought you were a nurse."

We'd already covered our careers when we had spoken on the phone, so he knew I'd been a teacher. "It just comes naturally after all the procedures my husband went through before he died."

"I could tell by talking to you on the phone that you were nice. That you cared about people."

Here we were, sitting on a park bench discussing health issues like an elderly couple while the wood nymphs frolicked beside us. We were at a stalemate. It was time for him to ask me questions to get the conversation going. Zack coughed and cleared his throat. "So, you were married a long time?"

This opened up a line of questioning that was dangerously headed toward suicide, but I was determined to avoid things ending on that topic. "I was married for forty-two years, until my husband got sick and died a few years ago." The last part of the sentence came out a little rushed, like I thought I might have revealed too much. We had talked easily on the phone about everything from the authentic dialogue in *Mad Men* to electric cars. Now the conversation felt stilted, but I couldn't think of another topic.

"So, what about your relationships?" I continued haltingly. All he'd told me before was that he was single, and I'd just assumed he was divorced or never married. "How long have they lasted?" I didn't know what the protocol was regarding questions about past relationships, but it was something I wanted to know, and I was tired of trying to make small talk.

Zack sighed and produced a bottle of Extra-Strength Tylenol from his pants pocket. He shook out three, popped them in his mouth, and then took a long sip from his water bottle. "I was going to tell you this before we, uh, got too involved. I'm actually still married, but I'm separated. My wife lives in Maine."

"So you're in the process of getting a divorce?"

"Uh, it's a complicated story. She decided to go back about seven months ago because her daughter was convicted of murder and there was no one to take care of the grandkids."

Any relationship with Zack was obviously out of the question now. I'd had doubts about his illness, but this new info was mortifying. I'm stubborn, though, and I was going to find out what his intentions were. He didn't seem up to a threesome.

"Why didn't you go back to Maine with your wife?"

"The cold really bothers my jaw and besides that, I didn't lie to you. We really are separated."

"Right, Maine is pretty far from California."

Zack looked hurt. "That isn't what I meant. We really aren't involved with each other anymore, but, like I said, it's complicated. We can't get a divorce for financial reasons. Neither of us makes that much and we can't afford separate places to live. Right now she's staying in her daughter's house with the grandkids."

"So how would I fit into this picture?"

"I thought that we could talk a little and get to know each other as friends."

"You don't go on online dating sites to find friends." My voracious curiosity forced me to continue pressing him. This meeting was like flash-forwarding through several seasons of *Days of Our Lives*, which Jean and I loved to make fun of.

"Then, who knows? When I get better we'd go out for a meal." Zack's smile turned to a wince, and he pressed his water bottle to his sore jaw. "I really gotta go now. The pain is getting worse."

I reached for Zack's hand. "Keep trying until you find the right doctor who can figure out what's wrong. You might have to leave the area to find one, but please don't give up." I surprised myself with this new concern for the health problems of others. If I'd met Zack under other circumstances, I probably would have kept in contact with him, maybe even tried to help him out. But we'd begun on one path playing the dating game and being a nurse to a very sick man didn't jive with my idea of male companionship. "Good luck," I said to him. Then I turned and walked out of his life.

I called Jean that night. "I'm oh-for-two." I told her about Zack's illness and weird marital situation.

Jean took it in with her usual informed platform. "There are a lot of men out there looking for a nurse and this guy sounds like he's actually looking for a *wet* nurse. But don't give up. You've just started. It takes a while to get into the groove. You have to be a bit of a risk-taker."

"No, I can't endure this anymore. Dating is too awkward, and it's hard to talk about my life without reference to Don," I said. "I'm now officially offline."

"This was just one experience. Maybe it's still too early, but someday you're going to find out how lonely it is out here."

I'd seen how some women changed when they began a new relationship. How some even switched political parties to match that of their new men. I'd been on Jean for years to eat more vegetables and less sugar, and she'd only started eating healthier after dating some new guy who was a strict macrobiotic vegan. "He doesn't eat bananas because they're too yin," my sister said without an eye-roll. When the boyfriend eventually disappeared from her life, so did the kale soup.

Although I would have been another person without Don's influence, I never changed to suit his taste. He never tried to convert me to Catholicism, and he accepted that I had "Christian values." It was as if we saw the things that mattered most through a unified perspective we had cobbled together through our years together. It made us a strong unit against adversity. We both distrusted the rich or those in pursuit of fortune and thought teaching was a more noble profession. Neither of us liked glamour.

We drove our scuffed and faded fifteen year-old-cars proudly in defiance of our friends and relatives who wasted their money on a new car before the old one had fifty thousand miles on it. Together we were always right. It wasn't as if I felt no one could replace Don, it was that I wanted to see how I perceived the world independently of someone else. The problem was I still felt frantic at the thought of being alone for the rest of my life.

Jean had a final bit of advice. "All of this could make a good book someday. Maybe writing about it will help?"

"A memoir about suicide doesn't sound very sexy. And I'm still living through it. I don't know the ending yet."

I thought of all the memoirs I'd read: Young women who go on journeys of discovery and face hardship only to find some sort of spiritual fulfillment and absolution in a happy ending. These memoirs were about survival. That's what people wanted, a story of how I fought the medical establishment and saved Don, not the morbid ending it was. I knew I wasn't carrying on in any heroic fashion using vodka to dull the guilt. No one would be interested in reading about a sixty-five-year-old widow who succumbs to alcoholism.

I did miss writing. It had been a daily part of my routine for fifteen years. I'd written nothing since I wrote the last words of my novel the day Don died. Writing was not going to heal me, but it might distract me and give me a focus.

Anna and I were sitting at the dining room table. I'd given her a short essay to read describing my online dating experiences and I felt proud of the writing. She was sewing fabric flowers on a fluorescent-green bra for an upcoming rave concert. I was happy that she was doing something fun. That we were both taking care of ourselves and each other. It had been almost a year since Don died.

I watched her face change from receptive to teary-eyed as she read; I'd hoped to make her laugh. "Why did you give me this?" she said.

"I thought it was humorous and poignant, the sort of tone I thought I wanted. I wanted you to see where I am right now."

"Where you are?" she said, nearly choking. "You want me to read this and say, 'Good job, Mom. I think this is very engaging'?" Her face was full of hurt and disgust. "What you're doing is trying to make a good story by exploiting Dad's death." She angrily wiped the tears from her eyes.

Anna was a woman who operated on a strict moral compass of behavior. She possessed a piercing sense of right and wrong and applied her principals rigorously to every phase of her life. When she was ten she announced that she was not attending church any longer because it was a sexist institution. In Catholicism, women had a lower status, and she couldn't abide by that. She was quick to jump on Don's case about stereotyping if he complained about "Asian drivers" when we got cut off by another car in traffic.

"I'm sorry," I said, trying to console her, but she batted me away.

"What I see here is you using suicide as a topic because you think it will make your memoir interesting."

"That's not it," I said even though she was partially right. I tried to manage a weak defense. "I just had to write, and this is how it came out." I realized I was mistaken in thinking my twenty-five-year-old daughter could also be my confidant.

"You said he blew his brains out. Why did you have to say it that way?"

"I can take that part out." I was looking for a way to deflect her, somehow squirm from black to a shade of gray. But Anna only thought in black and white.

"Go ahead and do your thing, Mom. But don't show me any more of this. And I don't want to know about you and these creepy men."

"I'm so sorry I did this. That I hurt you. Can't we talk about it?" I thought we'd become closer after Don's death. She had become withdrawn since she went away to college and it was puzzling to Don and me. One positive thing about Don's death was that it seemed that we had forged a new relationship. Last week she'd told me I was her best friend.

"I don't want to talk right now." She covered her face with her hands as if trying to block me out of her sight.

I'd made a huge mistake thinking she'd want to see where I was while she was grappling with her own emotions. We'd been down the same bumpy road but were now on different paths. I'd been focused on myself, and now I'd blundered and wounded her deeply.

"Now I have something else to feel guilty about."

I was still looking for Don to fill the void in my life and I expected Anna to understand, but Anna was looking for a father, a parental figure. She wasn't emotionally equipped to be a daughter and provide the support of a spouse.

Anna and I decided to do nothing at all to mark the first anniversary of Don's suicide. I had an appointment a week before with Doctor Perkin, who had known Don, but hadn't heard of his death.

"How is Don? Is he OK? I haven't seen him in so long."

"Don passed away about a year ago," I said. "As you know he had a bone marrow transplant about seven years ago, and he developed cryptogenic organizing pneumonia." I hoped that would end it.

"Pneumonia? Don actually died from pneumonia?" Doctor Perkin was not going to let it drop. He was a thoughtful and concerned man.

I looked across the doctor's shoulder at a poster showing the human anatomy. It reminded me of the drawing of Don's body as it was found that had been used in the coroner's report. I shut my eyes. "It's been a year," I said.

"So, I guess your family is probably going to have a special memorial for him for this anniversary?"

"No," I said. "He committed suicide. No one wants to be reminded of it, and we're certainly not celebrating anything about that date." The words shot out of my mouth.

Doctor Perkin looked shocked, but he'd asked for it. "I am really so sorry to hear that. Don was always so funny and upbeat. He was such a great fighter for his health."

"Yes, he was a fighter," I said. "That's the best way to remember him."

The anniversary of Don's death hit us harder than we expected. Anna and I both felt it coming weeks before the day arrived, but neither of us brought it up. The weather held up through October, and the beginning of November. California was still in a drought and we'd had no rain since April. Many of the shrubs on my property had not survived because I'd forgotten to water them. The supposedly drought-tolerant manzanita had lost their usual variegated green luster. The leaves from the deciduous oak trees had fallen into mounds three feet deep around my front pathway, blocking entrance to the front door. I started to let visitors in through the garage access to our house and passively watched the leaves pile up and the shrubbery die.

* * *

I called John on November 11, on the first year of Don's death. Aimée was in London visiting her parents and had texted and checked in with John all day. I was concerned that he was alone.

"I was fine until about an hour ago." His voice sounded shaky. "Then it hit me pretty hard."

"Me too," I said. "I didn't know what was going to happen, but the pain is still here." I regretted not driving up to San Jose to be with him, but that meant leaving Anna. She had professed no interest in talking to either John or me about Don, giving me a grim shake of her head when I'd asked her. John and I talked a little longer, and then emotion caused out voices to fade. We hung on in silence for a moment. I wished I could hug him. I wanted to say so much to him but couldn't find the right words to express myself.

I thought that I'd run out of all my options for recovery. Each time I tried to take a step forward, I retreated to even a worse state than before. Without Don as my sounding board, my mind went in any direction and my judgments were impaired. There would never be anyone who cared so much about me to take his place. I wasn't young and pretty anymore and, from the few conversations and "dates" with men, I felt inadequate to start in any new directions. If anything, I had less confidence in myself.

Chapter 10
The Cure Is the Culprit

Guilt was always there, in the understanding looks and sympathetic nods, when I discussed Don's death and the culpability of his doctors. Although no one said it to me, I knew there were questions about why I didn't do something.

Guilt was overshadowing grief. It was the joker appearing in my dreams, more pervasive than grief because it reached every part of my personality, entangled in my lack of self-confidence, lack of assertiveness, and lack of strength in the face of adversity. It decimated my character. Why did I refuse to have my dying mother-in-law move in with us? Why did I carry on a flirtation with a certain teacher and one of Don's doctors? Why did I abandon my father on his death bed when he asked me to stay?

It made me feel like I was a failure, not just in helping Don, but in my whole life. I knew this wasn't true—despite our separate ways of grieving, my daughter and I were close. And my son and I had grown closer, too.

Since Don had died, I'd awakened every night in a panic, remembering some incident in the past where I'd failed at something. Large incidents to small, they all vied for attention. I reviewed negative events—when I acted one way when I should have acted differently. My failures visited me from all parts of my life, from not helping a student in need to the look in Anna's eyes when she accused me of exploiting Don's death. All my flaws appeared in Technicolor. I felt the full emotional impact of the moment, trying to replay the entire scene and destroying myself in the process.

I remembered my mother visiting me at college to tell me that she and my father were divorcing. We were sitting in a restaurant, and her sandwich lay uneaten on her plate.

"Your father doesn't love me. He's going to leave," she cried.

I wanted to be anywhere else. I'd fled my family for a new life as a college student and now, here it was stalking me. "I don't know what I can do about it," I said. "I can't take sides." It was a cruel thing to say because I knew how hurt she was, and my sympathy would have helped her. But I didn't want to take on my mother's pain.

"I thought you'd understand," my mother cried. "That you, at least, would help me now." She was sobbing and her tears dripped down her cheeks onto her plate. I was alarmed, repelled by her emotional outburst and ashamed of myself for doing nothing to ease her distress.

"I have to go now," I said. My mother drove me back to my dorm. She was still crying when she drove away. I was glad I had no telephone in my room so she couldn't call me. A fissure opened in my mind and I knew this day would come back to haunt me.

My mother survived the divorce and came out better for it, but I wished so much she was still alive so that I could apologize for my appalling behavior. Before she died when I was thirty-one, I'd told her many times that I loved her, but it was not until now that I could feel her abandonment.

I was a bulimic, devouring and purging, powerless to stop this obsession with attacking myself. Each experience brought with it its own brutal self-therapy. I'd wake up at night with a fuzzy image of a past event, and then, like a photo from a Polaroid, the details became sharper until the entire scene played vividly and I couldn't turn away.

I dreamed about the last time I'd seen my father. I was twenty-four. He was in the hospital with congestive heart failure. I didn't realize he was dying since he had been battling this condition for two years. He talked about his disappointment at not getting a heart transplant. He'd been on the list, but his health had been considered too unstable to receive one. He looked weak and exhausted, his legs and arms thin and boney. I sat by the foot of his bed, anxious to go home after a day of skiing with Don. It seemed that my father had drifted off.

"I have to go now," I said.

He roused himself. "Can't you stay a little longer?"

I stood up. "I really do have to get back home." I didn't have to leave, but the tone of his voice scared me, and I feared having to face my emotions. It wasn't like him to plead. I left him.

The next morning the doctor called. "You need to come to the hospital," he said. "I have to talk to you about your father."

Don dropped me off at UCLA Medical Center and I ran down the hallway to my father's room. I was ready now for another conversation. Another man was in my father's bed. I stumbled backward and ran to the nurse's desk.

"Where's my father? He was in room 202. Where did you move him?"

The doctor came up then and pulled me aside. "I'm sorry, but your father died last night. I tried to get him to call you when he knew it was coming soon, but he didn't want to."

"Why didn't you call me if you knew?"

Don was there now beside me and took me in his arms. He led me away from the curious scrutiny of the crowded hallway. "Oh no," I cried. "He wanted me to stay with him and I left. He died alone thinking I didn't care."

I'd felt no sense of catharsis or relief with any of the therapies I'd tried, except the blotted temporary relief from drinking. I hated the word *grief* because it meant nothing to me. I wasn't sad and I wasn't tearful: I was full of blame at myself. I hated the "advice" offered from books, self-help groups, and friends.

As for therapy? Better to act like I was moving through the stages just fine rather than enduring another round of generic, one-size-fits-all advice. If an actual grief therapist didn't get it, then who would?

I knew I was still drinking too much. I even caught myself reaching in the cupboard above the stove for the cheap Gallo Vermouth I used for cooking when the other alcohol ran out. By the time I succumbed for a night of fitful sleep, my speech was slurred and my gait wobbly. I didn't think Anna noticed but she later made a comment that I didn't remember things she told me when I'd been drinking at night.

I saw how easy it was to become accustomed to having a drink by your side. I didn't start until sunset when the day had lost its focus and the night slammed down to hem me in. During the day I could escape by hiking, cycling, or going to the gym. But no matter how good the day had been—how full of the brilliant hues of friendship and activity—the night waited for me.

The bottles accumulated in the recycling bin, sometimes up to seven wine bottles a week and a liter bottle of vodka as well. When the trash truck came on Tuesdays and hoisted up my recycling container I could hear the tremendous clatter of the bottles crashing and breaking into the bed like a disapproving comment for the whole neighborhood to hear. Before, my recycling consisted of mostly of the tinkling of cans and newspapers.

I had to do something to distract myself to avoid drinking at night. Then a rash of emails arrived in Don's account from an online support group he had joined for people experiencing complications after their bone marrow transplants. They'd endured GVHD of the lungs, mouth, gut, liver, and skin and spent years living on 20 percent of their lung capacity. They had muscle cramps and spasms, neuropathology in their feet, painful skin tightening, and scoliosis. They used acronyms like AVN, PCT, SCT, and ECP treatments. We spoke the same language.

I connected to these people, patients fighting for their lives under similar circumstances as Don. They didn't want pity, they wanted just to have someone listen who understood, really understood what it was like to function on 20 percent of your lung capacity, how you could barely get out of bed each morning.

> Was wondering if anyone else with GVHD of the mouth has had teeth issues? My teeth have started chipping away.

> The GVHD in my eyes is going to make me claw my eyes out.

> I have developed severe cramping in my stomach. I was actually hospitalized due to high liver enzymes.

I posted Don's story, which I'd rehearsed and refined so succinctly over the many months since his death. Since most patients with GVHD are on prednisone, I intended only to warn about the dangers of the drug.

> Hi All,
>
> Here's my story. My husband, Don, a bone marrow transplant survivor for six years, committed suicide on November

11, 2013, while on the drug prednisone. This is a warning to all of you to please, please get yourself or your loved one under the care of a psychiatrist while on high doses of this drug.

Don was diagnosed as psychotic while on high doses (160 milligrams daily) when he was diagnosed with GVHD right after his BMT in 2007. He sank into depression after the dosage was decreased. I took him to a doctor, who put him on to antidepressants. He seemed to bounce back to his pre-prednisone self.

In May 2013, Don was diagnosed with pneumonia related to GVHD and given prednisone again. This time it was 90 milligrams a day. Don became manic, violent, and aggressive. I believe his symptoms suggested bipolar behavior. We live two hundred miles away from Maynard Hospital, where he was a patient under the care of the BMT team. I talked to his doctor there about my concern, asking for her to hospitalize him or get him psychiatric pharmacological help. She refused saying they were taking him off prednisone and he should be fine. She agreed that Don was "scary" and not himself.

As most of you know, prednisone of such high doses for a long period of time requires tapering. After about a month, when Don was down to about 10 milligrams a day, I noticed that he became very quiet, but I did not suspect he was in a dangerously suicidal state. If he had been under psychiatric care, it would have been noted because of the knowledge of the dangers of the drug by psychiatrists.

The weekend before his death, Don told me he was seriously depressed. The next day I started calling psychiatrist's offices to see if he could get an appointment. During that time, he left the house without telling me where he was going. It turned out that he drove to a nearby state park, where he took his life.

So, what is to be learned by this? Don was a fighter and advocate for his health. There is no way he would have taken his life under normal circumstances. His last visit to the doctors at Maynard was very positive in terms of his physical health. He was, in fact, considered the BMT patient "poster child." Now, after this incident, there is a psychiatrist on the Maynard BMT team, but I have to ask why it took so long? Why did my own psychiatrist tell me that Don should have been hospitalized during his manic phase and that there is no doubt that prednisone was the cause of his depression?

The responses came quickly, within the hour, from others who had gone through similar experiences. Instead of pouring another glass of wine, I read the replies.

My story is frighteningly similar to your husband's, except that I lived to tell the tale. I was on a moderate dose of prednisone for a lengthy period. I became slowly disassociated from reality . . . I became depressed. Wouldn't get up, wouldn't eat. This became so bad that one day I decided out of the blue to take a bottle of sleeping pills. Just before I lost consciousness, I told a family member what I had done. He called 911. I was brought back to life in the ambulance.

Contrary to Dr. Lin's claims, Don was not alone. The responses continued throughout the night and for the next week.

I was a caregiver for a friend who also underwent a transplant at Maynard in 2007, during the same time Don was there. A psych evaluation was required pre-transplant, and all sorts of pseudo-supportive statements were made about the psychiatrist being available after the transplant. When the need became a reality, the response was, "Oh, the psychiatrist doesn't take your insurance. Why don't you try the County Health Department?"

This person was referring to someone who had been treated at the same hospital, with the same BMT team as Don. Might have even been in the clinics with him at the same time, although we never met.

Dr. Lin must surely have known about this patient's mental problems and attempted suicide when she told me that she was unaware of suicidal behavior on prednisone. This patient had been at Maynard Hospital being treated by one of her colleagues. I knew the BMT doctors met every week to discuss their patients' progress. There was also the comment about a psychiatrist being available, so why had Dr. Lin told me that one was just now joining the BMT team?

I took the greatest solace in the words from strangers, who empathized in a way no one else could.

> I was admitted to the psych ward at John Hopkins after becoming extremely paranoid and delusional on prednisone. I am not even sure I would have gotten any treatment without the insistence of my wife. There were no psychiatrists on the BMT team and the GVHD doctor said he had never heard of psych problems on prednisone.

The last sentence was astounding. It was unbelievable yet horribly validating that someone had heard the same words. *The GVHD doctor said he had never heard of psych problems on prednisone.* At the same time, it was hard to read about this man being saved from possible suicide by the insistence of his wife. Unlike me, she had acted on her own and her husband was alive.

> When I had a flare-up (of GVHD) and they put me back on 60 milligrams (of prednisone) I needed to see a psychiatrist. Something was going to break: my sanity, my marriage, or one bad choice. Thank you for sharing this as not one doctor thought I needed or suggested me seeing a psychiatrist.

Another email arrived from the support group.

> At my last appointment with my BMT doctor, he asked if I would be interested in leading one of the BMT support groups because of my positive attitude. When I asked why, he said there had been recent patient suicides. Yes, his exact words.

A support group for prednisone depression without a trained leader was a Band-Aid fix. What a meager response from a highly trained doctor. It was becoming clear that Dr. Lin wasn't the only one who didn't take the devastating emotional side effects of prednisone seriously enough. Other doctors like her weren't doing anything to monitor their patients on prednisone. It was like giving a child an AK-47 with no instructions other than how to pull the trigger.

Forty more emails arrived. I sent ten of them to Dr. Lin with a note asking for her plan of treatment for monitoring patients on prednisone. This would be my therapy, a call to action, and I was sure she'd respond positively. She would be alarmed after she'd read the responses from the support group, and together we'd construct a plan. Lives would be saved, and my personal torment would end.

Dear Dr. Lin:

The day after Don's suicide you said that the Bone Marrow Transplant unit at Maynard Hospital and Clinics now had a psychiatrist working with the team to assist with mental illness evaluations for patients on prednisone. I have a few questions related to that, which I would like you to consider:

1. How available will the psychiatrist be to the many BMT patients you have on prednisone?

2. What is your plan for the psychiatrist? In what way will s/he directly assist patients?

3. What is your plan for monitoring patients who live great distances from Maynard like Don did? Will there be a Maynard affiliate in charge of the monitoring?

4. What is your plan for informing patients and caregivers about warning signs of mental illness and how to react?

Also, I wanted to refer to a statement you made to me during the same phone conversation we had the day after Don's death: "No BMT patient on prednisone has ever tried to commit suicide before." I have included emails I received from a GVHD online support group that indicate the common reaction of depression and suicidal thinking on high doses of prednisone. In these emails you will also find references to actual attempted suicides, including a patient from Maynard Hospital who was denied psychiatric help because the contracted psychiatrist did not take her insurance.

I have attached references to research studies about the connection between prednisone and suicide, which have appeared in peer-reviewed journals conducted by medical doctors and pharmacologists. Many of the reports suggest treatment plans using psychotropic drugs for severe cases.

While I blamed Dr. Lin for not prescribing medication for Don, I thought that she had acted out of ignorance. After she was enlightened by my email, I was sure that Dr. Lin would help me spread the word about prednisone. I also asked what conferences I could attend, what journals to submit to? I was on my way toward accomplishing a radical change in medical policies.

I waited for a week, a month, four months, and I received no response from Dr. Lin. I sent a follow-up email, but nothing came back except an automated reply that "Dr. Lin will be out of the office until January," which was three months away. She was ignoring me. My last hope faded and dissolved into another bout of guilt.

I fell backward even further into self-recrimination when I realized my instincts had been wrong again. Why should the doctors champion my cause when it would look like they made a mistake? Why would a prominent bone marrow transplant specialist from one of the world's top university hospitals listen to me about making a change in policy?

Don was collateral damage, his death the unfortunate result of the failure of the side effects of a drug. The doctors weren't responsible for what happened to Don, and they certainly weren't interested in maintaining any relationship with his widow. I needed to send them a stronger message, something to shake them into recognizing me. I had to make them acknowledge their responsibility.

Chapter 11
The Battle

I thought it would be easy. There were so many medical malpractice attorneys advertising on the internet: "If you or a loved one was injured due to the negligence of a healthcare provider, contact a law firm that puts families first. Call for a free consultation." I was on my way to a new beginning, to beating back the demons that crept into my dreams. Confident that any lawyer would see the certainty of a wrongful death conviction, I sent emails and made phone calls to their offices. I fantasized about my lawyer, his or her character a composite of Michelle Obama and Hillary Clinton. I read news accounts of huge malpractice awards, millions of dollars to families of victims. I would tell Don's story and lay out the facts surrounding his death. The evidence was there for any judge and jury. I speculated about how I'd spend the money—give enough to my son and daughter to pay off their student loans, travel the country speaking about the need to monitor patients on drugs like prednisone.

My calls were not returned, and I learned why when an attorney finally did call me back. I heard a dog barking and the metallic chirping of birds in the background. I imagined him at home, on his patio, taking the time to call me after a busy day.

"My firm can't take you on Mrs. Stegman, as much as we think you deserve it. California law only allows two hundred and fifty thousand dollars awarded to families for pain and suffering. If your husband had still been employed, we could get more for lost wages. Two hundred and fifty thousand won't even bring this case to trial." He sounded tired. "You don't want to do this anyway. Lawsuits are long, and they take you away from your family." The lawyer was waiting to get this phone call over. Waiting to get back to his family.

"And the low payment isn't the biggest problem. In order to prove that the doctors were responsible, your husband would have had to been actually in a psychiatric unit in a hospital under the supervision of doctors."

I couldn't believe that the legal system wouldn't support me. "I told the doctors that Don was mentally ill and they did nothing for me," I said. "How can they prescribe prednisone and not be responsible for what it does?"

"You have a terrible story, but we can only take on those cases we know will stand up in court. Even if this case made it to trial, juries are notorious for siding with the doctors. So we'd have that battle."

Every firm that bothered to contact me echoed the same opinion. The stories I'd heard of the "little guy" challenging unjust institutions and winning were flukes. The masses weren't rushing to my defense. The idea of justice for someone like me against Maynard Hospital was a fantasy I'd conjured up from movies.

I mentioned my intent to file a lawsuit to everyone when the subject of Don came up. No friend, family member, nor acquaintance missed my long discourse about how Don's doctors failed to intervene when they might have saved him. This provided fuel for my recovery. It also distracted me from my buried emotional discharge that still lurked beneath. Anyone who questioned my actions against the doctors was struck silent by my icy glare. Nor did I tolerate hearing, "Just let it go, Jill. It will be too stressful you or your family. You need to work on healing."

"You have no idea what grief is or what I'm going through." Anger is a potent defense against guilt. I was sure I was right and that justice would prevail.

John, still in law school, was the recipient of many of my questions. I deferred to him on all things legal. He came up to visit with Aimée whenever he got a chance.

We walked together on the beach arm-in-arm one afternoon nearly a year after Don died. It was low tide and the sand was firm under our bare feet. John's small King Charles spaniel zigzagged ahead of us, sniffing for sand crabs while Aimée tried to keep him from getting swept away by the incoming waves.

One thing that made me happy was the relationship John had with his wife. They had met and fallen in love when they were only twenty, the same ages as Don and I had been. They got married at twenty-four. Although she never complained, I knew it was difficult for Aimée: John was so busy with law school and her family lived in England. I knew that she'd take care of John better than I probably could.

I only watched war movies, and I'd seen *Saving Private Ryan* again. The heroes reminded me of Don and kept me pumped up about his case. I imagined speeches I'd make in court once my case came to trial. John asked me what movies I'd seen recently.

"I saw *Braveheart* and *The Deer Hunter*," I said.

"You never used to like war movies, especially when the hero dies," John said. "I watched those with Dad at home when you were gone."

"What do you mean?" I shouted above the surf. "I loved *Saving Private Ryan*."

"That's true," John said. We watched the surfers cutting through the waves for a few minutes, and then John turned to me again. "So what books have you read lately?"

"I just finished a really interesting book called *Lone Survivor*," I said. "It's about a Navy Seal who was the only survivor of a reconnaissance mission in Afghanistan."

John sighed. "I'm a little worried about you, Mom. Why are you so fixated on war and death?"

I thought for a minute while we darted out of the way of the incoming tide to a drier spot. "I guess it's that the protagonist reminds me of Dad."

John looked confused. "Really? Dad was never in a war."

"I know, but Dad had that drive and compassion, the all-out, bigger-than-life determination to do what was right."

John nodded. "I see what you mean."

"That's the way I feel about this lawsuit. Don't you think that's a good thing for me to do for Dad?"

John hugged me. "If it makes you feel better, then it is a good thing." He rubbed tears from his eyes. "I just don't want you to be disappointed. If you find an attorney, it's going to be a really long haul and that's going to be hard on you win or lose."

"You don't have to worry about me. This is what I have to do. I want to fight. It's what's getting me through this ordeal. I'd feel worse in five years if I hadn't tried everything."

This sense of righteousness empowered me to keep calling lawyers until I found David Eaton, who called back, saying he wanted to represent me. "I can hang my hat on this case," he said enthusiastically, which made me think I'd found the right lawyer.

Eaton's office was located across from the San Luis Obispo County Courthouse. His suite was behind a neo-Colonial sparkling-white building with a fountain in front that I now realize was actually a glamorous façade, as I had to follow a path leading past the front offices to an alleyway and up the back stairs to reach the law office.

He was overdue for a haircut and his red hair stuck out at clownish angles. He didn't fit my stereotype of a carefully groomed and polished attorney. Maybe his appearance was a deception to disguise a brilliant mind.

Eaton explained that he had spoken to a forensic psychiatrist named Richard Addison who wanted to be our "expert witness."

"I'm not sure what that is. I thought you were representing me."

"Malpractice cases like yours involving psychiatric issues are won or lost over the arguments of expert witnesses about whether the standard of care was breached and if the doctors should have done something more for Don when you asked them to help."

"And he wants to take on my case?" It was hard to believe that I was finally getting support.

"Yes." Eaton clasped his hands in mock prayer. "Addison is my friend and one of the best forensic psychiatrists around. I ran it by him and he insisted that we had a strong case citing the 'egregious' mistakes the doctors made in failing to get your husband psychiatric help when they had him on such a dangerous drug."

Eaton asked me for three thousand dollars up front to pay for Addison's initial report.

I balked. "I thought this was all on contingency."

"My fees are on contingency, but not the expert witness we have to hire. Doctor Addison will represent us against the other expert witness who represents the doctors."

"What would be the total cost I could end up paying? It seems like it could be a lot."

Eaton's enthusiasm was infectious. "It will probably settle out of court once they hear what Addison has to say. He thinks your case is very strong. The doctors should have helped out."

The Battle

I'd never spent money on something so intangible before. It was like gambling. I remembered that day Don died and the agony of the final realization that he had gone to take his life and would never return. If Dr. Lin had not ignored me I wouldn't be taking this step. I reasoned that nothing would happen unless I wrote the check.

I ordered medical documents from Maynard Hospital and everywhere else Don had been treated for the past seven years, which amounted to over a thousand pages of records. They came as a compressed file to download on my computer. Within these pages was the ammunition I'd need for my fight against Don's doctors. I saved a copy of the file for myself to prepare for battle.

Reading over the reports reminded me that when Don was at his sickest, we were the closest we had ever been. My role as his caregiver was defined. Don allowed me to take charge of him. Most of my energy flowed toward Don and his recovery. I'd rise in the morning and review what needed to be accomplished for Don. It was a grim time, but we were a team with a common goal. The day-to-day events were scripted by clinic visits, lab tests, pill consumption, and doctor's reports.

While my children attended classes every day and studied for exams fifty miles away, I counted out the pills and researched what they were for to arm myself for our visit to the clinic. Famotidine, sirolimus, amlodipine, clonidine, mycophenolate, prednisone . . . drugs to treat everything from heartburn to helping your body accept the new bone marrow as your own. There were drugs to treat viruses and infections that threatened Don's lowered immune system like moxifloxacin, voriconazole, and acyclovir.

Then there were the drugs used to combat the side effects of the other drugs like ursodiol to decrease the formation of gallstones and furosemide to reduce extra fluid in the body due to conditions such as heart failure, liver disease, and kidney disease. Haldol and Zyprexa for the symptoms of psychotic conditions. Ativan for anxiety.

* * *

I hoped that Dr. Addison would note that Don was only diagnosed and treated for prednisone psychosis after I dragged him into the hospital and he was given Haldol. I assumed that Dr. Addison would hone in on Dr. Lin's notes where she mentioned Don's depression during the five months after he came back home from Maynard:

> *October 2007:* Mr. Stegman was complaining of depression and unclear thinking and I advised him to keep exercising and look for volunteer opportunities.
>
> *January 2008:* Mr. Stegman's major complaints are those related to depression and emotion. He says that he continues to feel depressed and asked about when his life would return to normal. He was somewhat emotional but in no acute distress. We talked about him exercising more, including stationary bicycle riding.

Doctor Addison was reading this same report, and his conclusions must be similar to mine. It was clearly stated that Don had experienced prednisone psychosis before, back in 2007 when under the care of Dr. Lin. The records indicated the diagnosis and the prescription. The proof was undeniable.

I couldn't believe how Don was described in Dr. Lin's medical reports from that time because I knew he was not himself. He was lost and confused. He was still on many drugs including 90 milligrams of prednisone, as well as Ambien and Haldol. The medical records indicated about twenty different drugs in all.

I'd had to return to teaching in October 2007, since I'd used up my sick leave. I'd switched to teaching independent studies on a one-on-one basis to be more available for Don. He called me one day at work. He'd tried to use my debit card at the bank to get money and was refused. He wanted me to talk to the bank teller about it.

"Where is your debit card?" I said.

"I don't know. I guess I lost it." His voice sounded flat and distant.

He called me at my office again a few days later. I was with a student, so he left a message with the school secretary. "Don said that he's lost his car key down at the park, and you need to call him." It was the second key he'd lost, our only spare.

The Battle

When I got Don on the phone, he seemed panicked. "I don't know how it happened. I was taking a walk and the key must have slipped out of a hole in my pocket. Can you come and get me?"

"I can come and pick you up during lunch, but what are we going to do about the key? That was our only one. We'll have to go to the dealer to get another one."

"I just won't drive anywhere. It's what I deserve for being such an idiot."

We got another key, but Don still refused to leave the house. Sometimes I'd return home to find him napping, something he never did before. He became lackluster about safety—refusing to wear a seatbelt, getting cut with knives and saws.

I imagined Doctor Addison nodding to himself at the accumulating evidence of negligence. I poured my one-a-day only glass of cabernet, secure in the notion that by gaining justice for Don, I'd earned this reward. I was marked for special treatment by the universe and now my guilt would dissolve.

Chapter 12
Fault Lines

In September 2008, nearly a year after his death, I celebrated Don's birthday by inviting his brother Joe and his sister Teri to a barbecue at my house. Joe's wife, Bev, was there as well as Teri's partner, Natalie. Anna and Jean rounded out the group. I talked about the lawsuit, pretending not to notice their distracted responses.

"Eaton has sent out the preliminary letter to Maynard," I said to the group. "And the forensic psychiatrist is looking over Don's medical records."

"Mazel tov," said Jean, lifting her wine glass to me.

A week later Eaton summoned me with news back from Dr. Addison. I envisioned a hearty welcome and encouraging news that Don's death was due to gross negligence. When I'd first met Eaton, his disheveled appearance seemed quirky. But today he barely glanced at me when I walked in, looking rattled and confused, as if he had forgotten who I was. This time I noticed the chaos. Cardboard boxes with files and documents covered his desk and the surrounding floor space. He flitted over to an adjacent box and plucked out a file with my name on it. He sat back down and rubbed his forehead as he leafed through the pages. I sat across from him at the antique trestle table, the only nice piece of furniture in the room. I'd felt confident walking in, but Eaton's reception and weird confusion made me nervous. I sensed it was part of his lawyerly act to set a negative tone.

He finally found my file and withdrew a document. He plunked down heavily into his chair as if to forewarn me of the bad news coming.

"Dr. Addison isn't very positive about our case," he said. "He thinks the medical records indicate that the Maynard doctors were trying to save Don's life."

"But they didn't intervene," I said.

"They were tapering him off the prednisone."

"I know they were." I could hear the anxiety in my voice, but I managed to subdue it in order to act assertively, not defensively. "I know they weren't being callous. The point is they should have called in psychiatric help for Don, like I begged them to do. He needed it before, in 2007, when he became psychotic on prednisone. It's right there in the records. Dr. Addison must have read that. My own doctor told me that there was no doubt in her mind that Don's depression was caused by the prednisone."

"That's the other thing going against our case," he said. "The defense will jump on the fact that your psychiatrist was unprofessionally diagnosing your husband without seeing him, and you filed a lawsuit to cover your own guilt for your responsibility in your husband's death."

He'd said the words he knew would get me. My guilt. I tried to push away the paralyzing thoughts that came to me at the mention of that word *guilt*. People had to know that my guilt was separate from the doctor's guilt.

"I don't understand why it matters who influenced me to sue the doctors." I tried to keep the pleading tone out of my voice. I had to think clearly. "The point is they were negligent."

It seemed that Eaton had turned against me. "You knew your husband was suicidal. You said he was depressed the last week. They'll say you felt responsible that you didn't call the police earlier."

"I didn't know he was suicidal. I never said that anywhere. Did Dr. Addison actually read what I wrote down?"

I'd been naïve to think that I would get some closure on Don's death, prove to myself that I did all that I could.

"I didn't know what was wrong with him," I said, my voice rising. "I just knew he was mentally ill in some way so I asked for help. I didn't put together all of what the research said about suicidal behavior until the day he died, when it was too late."

I knew what was in the thousand plus pages of medical records dating from 2007 to November 11, 2013, because I'd read them all. Eaton had taken me on as a client based on what I told him was in the records. They demonstrated hospitalization and treatment for "prednisone psychosis" in 2007 followed by severe depression treated with Celexa. But none of that mattered. In the end, it would all come back to me and my culpability.

"I don't know what has happened to change your mind," I said, in what I hoped was a reasonable tone. "Only six months before Don died he was administered high doses of prednisone, up to 90 milligrams a day, and he became manic and violent. He wouldn't seek treatment on his own, so I'd contacted his doctors to give him psychiatric help. They acknowledged that he was not himself, but they refused to give him any medications. They said that tapering off prednisone would work. They didn't recognize his bipolar symptoms nor take his perilous mental state seriously enough. He committed suicide two months later. I don't see how that shows they were trying to save his life."

I continued to press my case. "What about all those studies that issued warnings about the high incidence of suicidal ideation in patients on even forty milligrams a day of prednisone?"

Only two months before, Doctor Addison had said to Eaton, "I think you have a very good case for a malpractice suit against the Maynard doctors."

What had made him change his mind?

"So, Dr. Addison thinks Don's doctors will be seen as heroes trying to save his life and *I'm* the one making egregious claims blaming them for his death," I said. "They'll turn the tables on me."

Eaton pulled out another piece of paper and studied it for a few moments. "They'll put you through hell. I've seen it and I know you don't want to go through with it."

I waited for Eaton to look up before I spoke. "They've already put me through hell. If I'm feeling guilty, it's because they put me here."

Eaton put my file down and walked over to his computer. He cleared off a stack of papers sitting on his printer. "What I can do is file a Letter of Intent. This will put the doctors on notice that they have committed malpractice, and that you intend to seek compensation. Then they have ninety days to respond."

"Then what?" I said. "It doesn't sound like you want to go through with this, so what's the point?"

"Who knows," Eaton shrugged. "They might just settle."

"Based on what you just said, isn't that unlikely?"

David Eaton, my savior, was bullshitting me. He'd given up on me. Looking out his window and across the alley, I could see the back of a meticulously restored Victorian home with its perfectly trimmed rose bushes and sculpted hedges, which housed the law offices of Burns and Stanley, the medical malpractice lawyers who did not take my case. I already saw the scenario played out, but I nodded anyway.

I took a wrong turn out of Eaton's office and got lost in a hallway that dead-ended in the office of a financial planning service. The receptionist must have seen that I was distressed because she walked me back to the door that clearly said EXIT.

Dr. Addison had read the medical reports but had decided that they supported the doctors. What I saw as proof of negligence, he'd seen as vindication of innocence. What was worse was that I'd be painted as the guilty one trying to blame the doctors when I could have stopped Don's death.

We got a letter from the Maynard attorney three months later saying she denied the claims I made against Dr. Lin and Dr. Major. "Mr. Stegman's psycho-emotional status was routinely followed with each visit by both of the above-mentioned providers." There was no mention of my pleading with the doctors to get psychiatric help for Don. "Maynard Health Care stands by the professional and personal actions of both of our providers; we assert that all of their care, communications, and actions fell within the standard of care."

An email came from David Eaton, detailing his doubts about the strength of the case, including the lack of documentation of my conversation with Dr. Lin when I asked her to prescribe medication for Don during the time he was so violent and irrational. Also included in the email was an additional charge from Dr. Addison of $755, which was for the additional hours he'd spent beyond the original $3,000 I'd given him. I called Eaton and demanded to get a written report from Dr. Addison or at least have a conference with him about his findings, but Eaton told me that, at $400 per hour, I probably wouldn't want to pay for a write-up.

"I looked at the billing that Dr. Addison sent," said Eaton. "And I think his charges were not out of line for the hours he put in."

"But I'd like him to at least explain to me what he saw in the medical reports that I didn't," I said. "We read the same thing, but he changed his mind radically from the beginning."

"It's not that he blames you," Eaton said in a soothing voice. "Dr. Addison looks critically at how the case will play out in court, and it's really tough to prove that a doctor is negligent."

I'd dreamed of making an emotional appeal to a jury, and how they'd be swept away by the details. The angry outbursts. My plea to the doctors to intervene. Don telling me that he was afraid of his thoughts, and then his body found at Whale Rock Reservoir. *Where I thought he would be?* Was that why Dr. Addison assumed I'd known that Don was suicidal and that I felt guilty because I didn't act soon enough? I'd written this all out in a preliminary statement to Dr. Addison when he asked for a detailed account of the last two weeks Don was alive. It should not have taken $3,755 of his time to conclude that I had no case.

It was December 2014, about a year since Don died, and one more pathway toward my vindication had closed. I wandered through my days in a muddle of conflicting emotions. Anger at Eaton and the unjust legal system. Humiliation at the tone of the letter in the denial of my claim: "If Mrs. Stegman had significant concerns regarding Mr. Stegman's wellbeing on November 11, 2013—they were not expressed to Maynard Health Care, Dr. Major, or Dr. Lin."

I sent the letter from the Maynard attorney to John and we talked about it on the phone.

"The letter pointed out only what I said regarding Don's actual suicide, not the fact that I'd asked the doctors for help when he was psychotic."

"That's right," John said with his usual patience. "That's because you're filing a wrongful death malpractice. You're saying that your husband is dead because the doctors were negligent, and the doctors are saying they had no clue that Dad was suicidal."

I persisted in my argument. "But they should have realized that he had a strong potential to be suicidal," I said. "All of this research I found says that patients on high doses of prednisone should be monitored, and he'd been psychotic and depressed before to the point of having to take medication."

"It's hard for most people to understand how the legal system works. The attorney's task is to defend their client, so they'll try to focus on one aspect of the accusation and distort its importance to show their client's innocence."

"There's all this other evidence, though, that could be used," I said. "The Maynard attorney mentions nothing about the conversations I'd had with Lin and Major about Dad needing psychiatric intervention. What really made Eaton drop me?"

"I'm not a medical malpractice attorney, but my educated guess is that Eaton thought, at first, that your case was a slam-dunk. That he could settle out of court, which would be the most cost effective for him considering he was doing this case on contingency, and he'd gotten you to pay Addison's costs. When he heard what Addison had to say, he realized it wasn't going to be so easy, that it might go to court, which would take lots of his time and money, so he lost interest."

"I feel like an idiot for spending the three thousand dollars. I don't think Eaton did hardly anything but write two letters. He wasn't well informed about my case. I had to repeat a lot of background information during our appointments."

"But you've always been a fighter, Mom. I remember that when my second-grade teacher wouldn't refer me for the gifted program, you pitched a fit and demanded that I be officially tested by a psychologist."

"I'm glad you remembered that," I said. "Maybe I'm not such a wimp after all."

* * *

I had felt strong and valiant when I'd decided to sue the doctors. Now I'd slipped back to a weaker position, but also one of more understanding about myself and the way institutions work. I didn't have the power to challenge the medical establishment on my own; I needed an army.

Chapter 13
Standard of Care

It had been eighteen months since Don's death. His features were fading. I had difficulty bringing him to life, and it scared me because I didn't want to forget him or how much I loved him. If moving on meant such a melting away of a spirit and soul, I didn't want it.

The medical board was my last chance to get justice for Don. I'd filed a claim a year ago, six months after Don's death, citing Dr. Lin as negligent in her treatment of Don for not properly treating him when he became mentally ill on prednisone. I'd carefully referenced the pages in Don's medical records where he'd received medication when he became psychotic before, in 2007, which Dr. Lin had noted.

I spent my mornings reviewing the details again over my cup of coffee. One morning Anna came out of her bedroom and found me at my computer mumbling.

"You all right, Mom?" she said.

"I have to get this right," I said. "Do you remember me telling you about the time I told Dr. Lin and Dr. Major that Dad needed psychiatric help and they said no?"

Anna picked up the comic section of the newspaper. "Yes. I remember that you were really upset after you talked to Dr. Lin about Dad. But I don't remember exactly what you said."

What was important to me was that I'd asked Dr. Lin to intervene when Don became psychotic. I mentioned that Dr. Lin had agreed that Don was "scary," but that she refused to prescribe any medication or offer to refer Don to a psychiatrist. She agreed that Don needed to be off prednisone, but she decided that after he was tapered off, he would be fine.

A year had passed, and I'd maintained faith that my medical malpractice claim against Dr. Lin would come through in my favor. Everything else had fallen through—my big lawsuit against

Maynard had backslid into more guilt. I certainly hadn't made a splash on the dating scene. I'd gained twenty pounds, and I wasn't carrying it well. I couldn't stand to look at the swollen image of myself at the gym. From a side view, I'd developed an Alfred Hitchcock–like appearance.

I got my bike out of the garage and pumped up the tires. I had a difficult time even mastering that small task. It took me thirty minutes because I had trouble fitting the nozzle onto my tire valve and kept releasing air. The day was sparkling and alive with spring, and I was eager to see the lupines and poppies spread out on the dry hillsides. I headed to Santa Margarita and a road Don and I used to follow. It was strange to be without my partner. I felt uneasy on the road by myself. I would have to learn to embrace being alone if I wanted to enter the world. I could leave my house and all the business of my life behind.

The letter came from the Central Complaint Unit of the California Medical Board. It stated, "Following a complete and thorough review of your husband's medical records, our medical consultant was unable to establish evidence of a violation that would result in disciplinary action against Dr. Lin's license to practice medicine in California."

Like the letter from the Maynard attorneys, this letter did not mention any recognition of Don's prednisone psychosis or my plea to Dr. Lin for help with Don.

> "The medical records indicate that fifty-six months following the ABMT (allogenic bone marrow transplant), your husband developed severe pneumonia which was successfully treated with steroids, but which appears to have emotionally traumatized your husband based on his *fear of choking to death if the pneumonia progressed*. According to our medical consultant, the treatment provided by Dr. Lin was appropriate and within community standards."

Of course, my complaint against Dr. Lin had not been for her treatment of his pneumonia, but for her negligence in treating his serious psychological state on prednisone. All of Don's mental health episodes and depression had been ignored by the consultant in the report. The medical consultant had determined the Don's suicide was "based on his fear of choking to death" if he contracted pneumonia again. Why would someone in a healthy state commit suicide because of this fear when he had just heard from his doctor that he had fully recovered? I knew where the consultant had gotten the remark, from Don's suicide note itself. I'd sent the note to the medical board because I thought it supported my claim about Don's state of mind and his fear of prednisone, and now it was being used against me.

Even as I read the note over two years later, I knew that the man who wrote it was not my husband. The personality simply was not his. Maybe the words were not of a psychotic person, but they certainly weren't those in a normal mental state.

> I take full responsibility for what I am about to do. You could not have stopped me. You should feel no sense of guilt for my actions.
>
> I do this because I am anxious, fearful, and depressed about the medical problem I will face. I do not want to choke to death from COP (cryptogenic organizing pneumonia). I do not want some inoperable cancer. I cannot face more hospitalizations, more rounds of high-dose prednisone.
>
> I have lost my inner strength to deal with the fears and anxieties that have never disappeared. I have tried to bury them and stay optimistic. I was successful some of the time. I can't continue to do this. I feel emotionally exhausted and unable to find hope for myself in the future. I have had suicidal thoughts throughout this entire last battle with COP. I have kept them hidden . . . hoping I could overcome them and find a positive perspective. I admit defeat.
>
> The burden I leave you is inexcusable. The burden I leave our children is also inexcusable. I hope that each of you will find it in your heart to forgive me. No family could have put up with me better than you have. I feel ashamed and guilty that I will leave you all to cope with my last actions. Please do not hate me. I know that you will be justifiably angry. I am extremely sorry for the trauma that I will have caused.

The doctors thought they were guiltless. If anyone could have intervened, it must have been a more observant me. The response from the mental health community was that many factors reflect a decision to commit suicide. Don's note suggested an internal battle with the forces of evil. But what were these battles but unfounded, irrational fears of "inoperable cancer" that was not on the horizon nor ever had been, "more prednisone," which Dr. Lin had told Don and the medical consultant he shouldn't require, and "choking to death from COP," which Dr. Major had stated was 94 percent under control? Don was in excellent physical health the day he died, and he knew it.

People don't kill themselves when they have good news. People kill themselves out of despair and anguish, when the struggle becomes exhausting, the prognosis poor, the divorce final, the career ruined, the humiliation unbearable. They do not hear, "Good news, Mr. Stegman, your lung capacity has improved to ninety-four percent on the Advair so you won't have to be on prednisone anymore," and then decide that all is lost, and they are doomed to die choking to death from pneumonia.

The medical consultant had used Don's suicide note to determine his mental state at the time of his death. The point of my complaint was that Dr. Lin did not properly treat Don when he displayed psychological distress. There was no mention in the medical board's letter that Dr. Lin was aware of Don's mental state during those last six months or that I'd asked her to help Don. The conclusions the consultant made about Don's state of mind must have come from his suicide note. The only reason I included the suicide note was to show the link to prednisone, and there was no mention in the letter from the medical board that prednisone had made Don psychotic and depressed in the past. It was as if the examiner had purposely sought to exonerate Dr. Lin.

The medical board had completed its review. There was no hope of appeal. The letter concluded with:

"As the consultant found that the care rendered in this case did not depart from the standard of care, no further action can be taken by the Board. Therefore, no further review will be conducted and the complaint is closed."

What in the hell did "the standard of care" mean? According to the research and articles I'd read, Don's symptoms of psychosis meant that he should have been treated with medication or at least monitored:

"Educating patients and their families about these adverse events and increasing primary care physicians' awareness about their occurrence should facilitate early monitoring," write the investigators (Fardet, Petersen and Nazareth, 2012).

This letter used the same legalese language as the one from the Maynard attorneys, "no further action," and "no basis for the claims against Dr. Lin."

Even rereading the letters from the Maynard attorney and the medical board now, over a year later, was a surreal experience. I was filled with anger reading the vigorous denial of any wrong-doing on the part of the doctors and how they had succeeded so often in treating Don for his physical problems, brought him back from the brink of death. Parsed out in legal phrases, it was easy to see how manipulation and omissions can distort the evidence. Neither letter addressed the warnings from the research, Don's previous psychosis, or the fact that I'd asked both doctors for help.

Chapter 14
The Road to Recovery

The medical board may have thought my case was closed, but I was not finished. After all, this was not only about Don's death, but for the others who took prednisone to manage symptoms but instead had much scarier outcomes.

State Senator Katcho Achadjian's Sacramento office contacted me to say he'd be in San Luis Obispo in March. He wanted to meet with me regarding a proposal I'd sent to him suggesting that he introduce legislation requiring monitoring of patients on corticosteroids like prednisone. I'd emailed him Don's story, changing my tactic once more from attack to cooperation with the medical establishment. The general letter had the same damning sentences about prednisone minus the accusations of Dr. Lin's negligence. My suggestion for his forthcoming agenda was for better "monitoring" of prednisone and corticosteroids.

I was nervous the morning of my appointment. I'd never spoken to a state senator before, and I wondered about the protocol. How, exactly, would we interact? I pulled on a pair of black slacks and a conservative blue shirt. It was a uniform I'd worn to teach in and had served me well during those years. At least it never went out of style. I rummaged in the closet and found a dusty pair of silver pumps. I looked at myself in the mirror and saw that the shirt could have used a little ironing and the jacket needed brushing. I'd need to buy new clothes if I planned on future meetings to advocate for better monitoring of prednisone.

Senator Achadjian's field office was located on the fourth floor of an office building in downtown San Luis Obispo. Fully armed with files of the research studies to back me up, I took the elevator to the second floor and walked into an empty office. I heard murmuring down the hallway, and then a senior field aide appeared. His manner was polite but diffident. "Katcho is waiting for you;

please follow me." He led me past photos of the state senator shaking hands with officials at public events and fundraisers. The walls were plastered with plaques of support for his service to the community. I would tread another path. Maybe this was the man with the power, who would want to do the right thing. There were, after all, about twenty million people in the United States on drugs like prednisone.

Mr. Achadjian, a dark-haired, balding man with a mustache, was difficult to read. He smiled solemnly as he shook my hand and indicated a table where the three of us sat down. I waited nervously for him to begin the conversation, maybe ask me some general warm-up questions, give me a report, but he said nothing. Technically he had asked to meet with me, so shouldn't he start? The aide picked up a pen and wrote something on a yellow legal pad. They were waiting for me.

I'd rehearsed no opening comments, nor schmoozing remarks about life as a state assemblyman. My life and Achadjian's intersected only at this point, and I had no interest in casual conversation on any other topic.

"I know you have already read my suggestion about monitoring prednisone, but I wanted you to hear the events from me as I lived it." I'd explained and examined the details of Don's story so many times, and from so many different aspects, I simply began speaking in the pre-rehearsed, professional tone I'd adopted with the new slant on the importance of monitoring corticosteroids.

I heaped the facts of Don's experience on him, careful not to attack Dr. Lin or say anything about the lawsuit or complaint to the medical board. Finally, I pointed out my carefully highlighted research studies, "So you see, it says right here in multiple studies that doctors are overlooking the severe mental reactions of patients on prednisone, and that they should be monitored. There are twenty million people on prednisone in the United States." Achadjian had been silent the entire time I spoke, his hands clasped on the table.

"How long has it been since your husband died?"

"It's been two years now."

"I ask because I have a personal interest in your case. In what you're going through." He spoke with a noticeable accent, and I remembered that he's been born in Lebanon. "My mother was in the hospital for a simple surgery. When she came out of the anesthesia she acted very weird and disoriented. She was paranoid. She didn't know her family. The doctors and nurses at the hospital didn't know what was wrong. We finally got her GP involved who figured out it was a drug reaction. Who knows what would have happened if she'd been at home."

His words alone made me feel vindicated.

"I do support your idea of monitoring, and I have approached the two big sources we would need to be on our side to pass any legislation, the medical board and the insurance companies. Unfortunately, both of them are adamantly opposed to requiring any monitoring of prednisone."

I heard my sister's voice, "I can't believe you ever thought you could sue Maynard Hospital." Where was my counter balance? Couldn't the right thing prevail because it was just?

I still had to ask the question. "Why?"

"The insurance companies said it would be too expensive to get psychiatrists and drugs involved. The medical board said that there is a law which allows you to have someone committed for seventy-two hours if you think they are a danger to themselves or others. This is something you could have done for your husband."

Here it was again. It was my responsibility to monitor Don. "The medical board is saying that this is supposed to be something I could have done to save Don even though I didn't even know anything about it? Why didn't Dr. Lin tell me about it? Why didn't any of Don's other doctors tell me about it when I asked for help? Can't we get some kind of brochure to give to families that has this kind of information in it? You know, warning signs and steps to take?"

"That would be a good idea." Achadjian glanced over at his aide who dutifully wrote something on the tablet. They both looked at me. Did I have anything else to say?

"The insurance companies and the doctors don't want to enforce the monitoring so that's the end of it?"

"No, this is where the hard work begins. This is where we have to get support from consumer groups and other supporters to advocate. We have to show that enough people want this change."

I thought of my naïveté in thinking that people naturally wanted to do right by Don. That Dr. Lin would, of course, be eager to collaborate with me to demonstrate an improvement in monitoring patients on prednisone. That the medical board would consult with a mental health professional to assist on my case against Dr. Lin. And I'd envisioned myself in some heroic role passionately and eloquently convincing judge and jury of the negligence of Dr. Lin in not caring for Don's psychosis.

I knew that my cause would be diluted by the larger agendas of mental health and suicide prevention. I wrote to every institution and consumer advocacy group I could find, including Consumer Watchdog, and no one contacted me. The National Mental Health Association and American Prevention of Suicide wanted my money and volunteerism but weren't interested in lobbying for my specific cause.

Even for my failed efforts, I did not feel foolish, which was new for me. Through this process, I'd learned more about myself and the dynamics of grief. I'd instinctively fought for Don's honor for my recovery, not to blame someone else for my guilt. The decisions from the medical board and the legal establishment were against me, but their justifications were poorly determined and weakly explained. I had become experienced in the process of institutional change. I believed that institutions would protect me. I believed that justice would prevail. I don't know if advocating more strongly for Don could have helped, but I decided that I would not stand back anymore. If something didn't seem right, no matter where it was coming from— doctors, hospitals, or police—I was going to make a stand.

Chapter 15
Naked with Strangers

I looked for new avenues while I waited to be pulled in a new direction. What would it be like to begin again, to go backward in time? Up the coast near Big Sur was Esalen Institute, once known as a haven for the alternative lifestyle and New Age thinking. At the time of its inception, in the sixties, I'd laughed it off somewhat, believing the "free love" philosophy emanating from the place supporting co-ed nude bathing was more of a male-oriented interest in possible sexual encounters than anything to do with philosophical discussions. I knew that beyond the wild encounters was the legacy of Alan Watts and brilliant masterminds Michael Murphy and Richard Price, who'd ushered in the human potential movement that still resonated. I was a little late to the party, but I was ready to be transformed. I paged past the listed workshops on "Love, Sex, and Intimacy" and "Tantra, the Art of Conscious Loving."

I found myself at a week-long yoga class studying shadow yoga and meditation. At twenty-five I'd twisted myself into the various pretzel-like asanas with balance and grace, my slender body easily molded into a graceful tree or lithe model of a goddess, and I expected nothing less of myself at sixty-seven, even though I weighed an additional thirty pounds.

The first session began in the pre-dawn darkness, a large yurt filled with seventy-five yogis. This was no geriatric, post-hippie crowd. A quick glance around the roomful of figures revealed that I was probably the oldest. Shadow Yoga was not the "gentler, kinder" yoga I had known forty-five years ago. It involved more athletic, squatting postures, which is why it probably attracted these youngsters. At a gesture from the instructor, everyone but me dropped fluidly to a squat with their butts an inch from the floor. I spread my knees, went about halfway down, tried to ratchet my rear end down farther, and froze. Two assistants propped me up with pillows so that I could at least assume the position. From my ridiculous perch I thought, "This is only the first day; I will prevail."

After that session I ventured down to the baths, just to take a peek at those famous waters representing the era of newfound sexual freedom. Don and I had missed that calling, been loyal to each other. In that way, we were quite conservative. But, like many others of our generation, we lived together before we got married without revealing that fact to our parents. The lengths we went to covering up this transgression seem silly now.

The narrow path wound down the cliffside past a sign that read "No Unwanted Touching" and another, "Absolutely No Photography." The baths were set on promontories with the sparkling water beneath. I looked down on one bath and saw the shimmering torsos of two couples, slim and uplifted breasts and muscular pectorals. They were conversing like friends meeting in a park. I walked by with an awkward smile and turned back up the path. This full daytime exposure was too stark and revealing. Maybe I'd return at night.

I wanted to be more relaxed. I'd been swimming naked with strangers before with Don when we were in our thirties. I remembered practically nothing about the experience, definitely not feeling embarrassed or self-conscious. The Esalen brochure had stated that the baths were a place for "personal sanctuary and respect for the human body," something I'd keep in mind.

The afternoon meditation session consisted of chanting some words in Sanskrit about overcoming your boundaries and setting your intentions. The young voices sounded beautiful and heartfelt lifted in harmony. I chanted along with them rather disingenuously because I couldn't quite erase the image of Hare Krishnas from the sixties and seventies in their pastel robes begging at the airport, although these more modern devotees were much more sophisticated and educated than the lost souls I remembered from my generation. We faced the small statue of the elephant god, Ganesh, the remover of obstacles.

My idea of meditation from forty-five years ago was sitting in silence with someone guiding you to a higher level. Not exactly praying, which I knew wasn't me, but a search or quest. But here I was, chanting before an elephant god. I closed my eyes and opened my mouth in a soundless incantation, allowed the chant of the group to channel through me. The voices resonated, the feeling of community was powerful. By the end of the week I could inch down slightly closer to the floor in my squat and modify the other asanas.

I returned to the baths on the last night of the retreat. In the darkness I was just another inconspicuous figure. I found a small tub on the end, slipped out of my robe, and stepped into the water. The odor from the natural spring feeding the baths was mildly sulfuric. I found myself humming the chant we had practiced that week.

The stars and planets configured the sky and the ocean banged and sucked against the cliffs. Now I was alone, naked in this primordial setting hanging over the Pacific. This was exactly where I was supposed to be. I was sure of that. I could go back and find myself. I knew Don wasn't here with me, and that he never would be. One of my friends had insisted that someday Don would speak to me. Linda, from the suicide survivor's group, had said her son, Aaron, had spoken to her a year after he shot himself. I was happy for them in their faith, but I wasn't a believer. When I looked up and felt the embrace of the starlit sky, I was comfortable with the idea of oblivion. But the harshness of atheism and the vacuum and nothingness of the cosmos couldn't explain the sensual beauty of the human spirit.

When Don appeared in my dreams, he never blamed me for his death. It was always a realistic scene from life as I knew it. As I woke, I thought that it could have been a memory. We didn't have a perfect marriage. There were times we didn't communicate very well, when we probably could have used marriage counseling as we blasted, rather than molded, our way through our forty-five years together.

I learned more about our relationship and what love is really like after Don died. Suicide was my entry into self-analysis and rebirth. That is the suicide survivor's manifesto, to review and criticize. I'd told Don he was the most important person in my life. And he died knowing that. In a way the devil did get him, but he'd die before he'd let the devil get me.

Chapter 16
Slowing Down the Race

My life in review was a series of half-assed attempts and limited successes. I gave up on teaching after only one year. I gave up playing the piano after three years. Now the instrument sits in my living room, unused for thirty-five years except for a brief period when my daughter bashed out a cacophony of clashing chords at age six. I gave up on landscaping my property—one side of the driveway has native shrubs and trees, while the other side is bare of anything but gopher holes. I gave up on tennis and golf because I lost the motivation to practice.

Don might be alive now if I hadn't given up. I told his doctors something was terribly wrong with him after they prescribed prednisone for his pneumonia. His personality changed almost overnight to a violent and abusive stranger. I should have insisted to Don's doctors that Don be hospitalized because he was a danger to himself and others instead of accepting their dismissal of my concern and doing nothing. I sat by during Don's depression, missing the signs as he slumped deeper past a point of no return.

I wanted to challenge myself; cleanse myself of all the fighting and campaigning I'd been doing—to see if I could do something that maybe otherwise Don would have helped me accomplish.

The climb was far steeper than what was described in the brochure, a 20 percent grade of hairpin switchbacks twenty miles to the top. I looked down at the coast we had left a few hours ago, and the sea was a dim blue ribbon below at the base of the road zigzagging up like a bleached backbone of a giant reptile. I was more than halfway, in the forest now, but the swirling pines offered no respite, just a reminder of the elevation yet to gain.

The other riders were all women, which I thought would set a more moderate, less competitive tone. Our ages spanned from forty-two to sixty-seven, my age. I looked forward to the camaraderie of female companions, being single and with no man now or on the horizon. I thought that an all-women's tour would be less competitive.

I was proven wrong when, on the second day of riding, one of the forty-two-year-old youngsters, Ruth, tried to nudge me out of my lead position directly behind the guide. I refused to let her in because I was maintaining the pace right on the guide's tail. I glanced over at her with a what-the-hell-are-you-doing? expression. Was this the Tour de France? Were we supposed to queue up by age? Was I unaware of some rule of the road? Grim-faced, she dropped back into an open space. She'd get back at me later.

This is the last and hardest ride of the eight-day bicycle tour in Albania. When I signed up for the trip in May 2016, I was lured by the prospect of visiting an unspoiled country and riding untrafficked roads. The "rolling hills" described in the brochure sounded perfect for me. I pictured myself soaring along enjoying nature and forming an *esprit de corps* with the women.

The trip turned into a much different experience. The rolling hills were often hard climbs of thousands of feet. Yes, there was little traffic—because the roads were so bad, sometimes only patches of asphalt over gravel. And the competitive vibe changed what the trip meant to me. Over the course of a few days the ride became a quest. I made a commitment to myself to ride the entire time without getting picked up by the support vehicle to confirm that I'd changed. That I didn't give up when things got hard. That I was self-reliant. I could push myself to accomplish my goals. Mostly, that I didn't give up.

To my credit, I trained alone for this ride in "unexplored" Albania. For months I'd ridden up to forty-five miles a day on the "rolling hills" around my home on the central coast of California similar to the topography described in the itinerary. I felt prepared. But I'd only been on one climb like this, albeit much shorter, up Old Creek Road, which passed the place where Don's body was found. I originally went into the ride thinking I could always get a lift when I got too tired. Now I'd turned this into something else; I had something to prove. Making it all the way up the 3,400 feet was a way of climbing out of my old give-up-when-the-going-gets-hard ways to my new don't-give-up self.

I strained hard with each breath and had to dismount to rest for a minute. The support van nudged up to me, but I waved it on. It had been following me like a vulture waiting for an animal's last gasp. It moved on to the next pullout a few miles up. I'd had cortisone shots before I left, so my knees served me well. I'd done well on the previous days of riding, coming in among the first riders.

The day had been tough since we'd left the coast a few hours earlier, and I'd fallen farther behind. I was breathing hard and couldn't seem to get into a regular pattern. I kept coughing up mucus, throwing off my breathing even more. At first I cared about not being last, now I only cared about making the entire climb. Lunch awaited us at the top, a few more miles away, where I could enjoy the view and marvel at my accomplishment.

I had to make it because I wouldn't be returning to Albania, though it was a gorgeous country. We'd been following the border with Greece in a landscape of crimson poppies, sweet peas, and a spectacle of various shades of green. My dreams were a kaleidoscope of verdant images.

The sciatica on my left side produced a nagging complaint. A herd of sheep in the road gave me an excuse to dismount. The sheep swarmed across the road frantically, the dogs trying to bunch them together by nipping and bullying. I stayed clear of them all, flattening against the side of the mountain with my bike in front of me. The dogs would attack if I got among the flock. The sheep were mangy and tattered-looking beasts on their way to better pastures or a slit throat. No need for them to have fine wool. The sheep herder passed with a thick wooden stick he whacked on the back of a straggler. I grabbed my camera to get a shot of him and the sheep. It's a sight you don't encounter in the USA. I didn't think the shepherd looked at me, intent on his flock, but when I reviewed the photo later, I saw that he had glanced my way, smiling. A car approached, braking for the sheep, and then paused by me. The driver aimed his cell phone at me. Apparently, I was as much of an anomaly to him as the sheep were to me. My grimace might look like a grin when he showed it to his friends and family.

The hill was so steep that I was barely moving, and there was a shooting pain emanating from the left side of my buttocks. Any slower and I'd lose my balance and topple over, so I decided to walk awhile to relieve the ache that ran from my butt down my left thigh. The sheep had disappeared around another switchback. How many more switchbacks to the top? It would help to have a countdown. The sheep herder yelled from a distance and a dog yelped; maybe he got the wrong end of the stick for not doing his job.

Yesterday I'd basked in the Adriatic with the other women, and we had dined on delicious mussels and grilled zucchini. The water was warmer than the Pacific, so soothing after the previous day of cycling. When we left this morning, I'd looked up at this hill, and knew it had been my fate to be here, to test my endurance, mentally, physically, and spiritually. I was already testing myself physically and mentally and the results were still inconclusive, but ongoing. The spiritual test was yet to come.

A stone church jutted out on a rock precipice a hundred yards above me, affording another excuse to get off the bike. If I stood in the middle of the road and craned my neck, I could see the circular basilica and rooftop cross. These small Christian churches were ubiquitous in Albania, present in every neighborhood, even though the country was now over fifty percent Muslim. They were simple structures in the Eastern Orthodox style left over from the Byzantine era when Albania was mostly Catholic. I was fascinated with the neatness of the compact church structures and the simple icons of the saints with heads encased in golden halos. Some find the wooden expressions of the icons austere and emotionless. I was drawn to the focus on the eyes: black orbs radiating from their faces, entreating prayer not for forgiveness or intervention, but for perseverance. If I were religious, I'd join them. Their haunting eyes encouraged me to persevere in my own small way.

Don would have liked these churches. He had left Catholicism and its priestly trappings years ago, disavowing the idea of divine intervention after pulling through cancer on his own. He believed in a brand of humanism centering on individual strength of spirit. "We all have the tools to survive deadly diseases; we just need to learn to tap our inner resources." He was living proof of this for many years until the prednisone took over and altered that part of the brain which controls your perceptions and emotions.

The church hung above, inviting me to visit and sit a while among the saints. I imagined their frescoed images in the flickering candlelight. It's common for believers to light a candle or two before their favorite saint, asking for a special favor.

Raindrops tapped the surrounding foliage. I had climbed into a cloud, which meant there was only a short distance to the top. My group had probably already arrived at the lunch-stop and were ensconced by a fireplace warming up while I slogged it out who-knew how many miles away. I knew they weren't waiting for me. The van was somewhere ahead, but I didn't consider flagging it down. The only one who gave up? That wasn't going to be me.

I had no raingear and my lightweight wind jacket was plastered to my back. I packed for sun, for mild weather. My wet Spandex shorts began chafing my crotch. The support van was parked a few switchbacks away, but it wasn't raining that hard. I thought I could outride the storm if I focused on the road.

I cranked along in a trance until I shut down. The pain from my sciatica shot down my back. When I got off the bike, the pain floated away. When I got back on, it returned to the same intensity, like flipping a switch. The support van appeared, and I allowed the driver to pack my bike on the trailer. I climbed into the van feeling like a miserable failure. Fortunately, the driver spoke only Albanian, so I wasn't forced to make conversation. We drove about a mile to meet the others at the appointed lodge.

The other women ignored me when I sat down to lunch. Most of them had finished eating and were sharing stories of their glorious triumph. They were giddy with their victory. How hard this or that switchback was. How the climb compared to Bhutan or New Zealand. None of them passed the sheep or saw the church or noticed the trees. They were so intent on the goal or too miserable to notice. I was among them, but not of them, the only one who didn't make it the whole way.

We still had twenty miles to go, much of it downhill, but some short climbs over rolling hills. Everyone climbed back on their bikes. It was raining and chilly. Two of the women, exhausted, decided to ride in the support van. No one blamed them; unlike me, they made it to the top. The rest gathered their remaining strength for the finale.

I looked at my bike sitting on the trailer. No one was going to give me any street cred for making it 90 percent of the way. It was all or nothing. But I felt rested after lunch, and I really didn't want to get back in the support van with the other two dropouts. I knew that if I'd rested a little more, I could have made it. Our guide said it was one of the toughest climbs she'd ever been on, and she'd been cycling all over the world in all kinds of weather. I decided to ride the remaining miles. I knew I'd never feel the same way as the others, those who made it to the top, that I didn't "earn" a seat at their table, but it didn't matter. Something happened to me that the others didn't experience. I was all alone on an Albanian mountain for a while, but I didn't feel lonely. My senses were heightened, and I felt tuned in to the world. I wasn't done yet.

I signaled the driver and he unloaded my bike with a wink and a nod. I borrowed a rain jacket from one of the dropouts and climbed on my bike. The other women had taken off already down the steep slope, visions of a celebratory evening in their heads. They were a solid flock of winners.

But I had my own celebrating to do. Against the advice of our guide who had alerted us to the "dangerous road conditions," I sailed off, pedaling as fast as I could until I hit such a high speed I could only coast. I flew by a group of women who were tentatively dodging potholes. I braked slightly, my back tire thumped over a pothole, and I was practically airborne, but I had done this kind of riding twenty or thirty years ago when Don and I rode mountain bikes together. I instinctively focused on the road, anticipating what was ahead, zig-zagging expertly around the potholes and gravel like a skier working moguls. This kind of skill doesn't atrophy with age. The landscape was a green smear, beautiful or mediocre; it was irrelevant to me. I wanted to get down this hill as quickly as possible and be the first to the end. I didn't want anyone's admiration but my own.

I'd always been a wimp on the down-hills; my fingers cramped from grasping the brakes. Now I felt liberated, eager with anticipation. I passed more riders, two and three clumps of them at a time. The terrain flattened and a few riders were trying to give me a run for the money, but they couldn't keep up. I took the rolling hills easily, feeling fresh and strong. Finally, the lead guide was only yards in front, followed closely by the three strongest riders. I approached the group and passed all of them, including the leader who looked surprised. I didn't know if I'd committed a faux pas by passing the guide. Why shouldn't I? It was a straight shot to the hotel.

It felt good leading the pack. I knew I would have to pedal like a mofo to stay in front, that the lead guide could easily overtake me. He may have wanted a slower pace. He did pass me after a few miles, followed by the rat pack of three who refused to let me break up their triad. I was forced to ride behind them for the rest of the way or pass all of them including the guide; they were packed so close together. I couldn't go fast enough to pass them all and not quickly be overtaken. Ruth was the first behind the guide, determined not to let me in. The other two were locked into place like railroad cars, mouths tightly set. I could only follow. *I'm twenty-five years older than you are*, I wanted to scream. I fell off the pace and veered off toward the sea, taking my time to reach the hotel. I wanted to miss the jubilation, the comradely remarks about making it the whole way. What would I do but stand on the periphery?

I wasn't allowed to live out my pouty childish fantasy. The last two riders, the married couple, Marla and Laurie, saw me poised by the coastline pretending to take selfies with the drab offshore islands as a backdrop. They were worried about me.

"You were screaming when you went by us," said Laurie. "We thought something was wrong with your bike when we saw you over here."

I could have flagged down the van, but Marla and Laurie insisted on lending moral support. They had already become my favorites because of their easy confidence and noncompetitive spirit. Although they were highly skilled riders, with trim and well-toned athletic bodies, they took their time on the rides, preferring to hang back to shoot photographs or offer encouragement to other riders.

I thought they were just good friends until I'd asked Laurie what her husband did.

"I don't have a husband, I'm married to Marla." She held up her hand with the large diamond setting and Marla, sitting across from us, held up her hand with the identical ring.

They gracefully waved off my apology and wouldn't allow me to be embarrassed. Here were two women who were content in their own skin. Anyone could learn about relationships by observing Laurie and Marla's attention, care, and concern for each other while remaining independent. Laurie was on her way to Macedonia after this trip and Marla would be venturing to England to visit a friend.

The revelation of their marriage gave me even greater admiration for them. They had made something which sparkled between them and affected those around them like few other relationships I'd observed. I didn't think I would have realized this if I were still married. At that time my perceptions had been filtered through Don's vision. If I'd been married, I probably wouldn't be riding a bike through Albania or experience it the same way.

That evening, as the other riders recaptured their experiences and the rugged climb of our final day, I didn't feel that I'd failed. I'd ridden to exhaustion, and then, like the horseback rider who gets thrown and climbs back on, I'd rested a little and tackled the rest of the ride, going all out and being out front, alone, for part of the way. What I'd seen as failures in the past were only because I'd given up. Being alone had not terrified me, had not made me feel abandoned.

Epilogue

I continue to study the research on the importance of monitoring patients on prednisone with a focus now on bone marrow transplant patients, since they are potentially prescribed the higher doses for the longest periods of time. A 2011 study which followed 2,330 bone marrow transplant patients concluded:

> Those managed with prednisone for their chronic GVHD are at significantly increased risk for psychological distress. Prevention of the psychosocial consequences in the BMT survivors may be realized by interventions that help healthcare providers optimize the medical care for conditions such as chronic GVHD, as well as interventions aimed at helping them cope more effectively with the burden of illness. . . .
>
> The current study demonstrates that after a median follow-up of 7 years, bone marrow transplant survivors exposed to prednisone and the presence of active chronic GVHD were associated with an increased risk of reporting psychological distress. To reduce the burden of psychological distress in this population, specialized multidisciplinary management involving both physician and psychologist is needed (Sun et al. 2011).

There are hundreds of thousands of bone marrow transplant survivors who are still alive up to forty years after their treatment. Since Don had his bone marrow transplant in 2007, there have been approximately one hundred fifty thousand BMTs performed in the United States, and the survival rate is currently nearly 85 percent.

It was heartening to see that these studies had been published in well-respected hematological journals read by doctors performing in the field. According to the information on their websites, many hospitals and clinics listed specific plans for the long-term care they offered, including social and psychological services and annual evaluations.

Had Maynard actually done anything in the five years following Don's death to help patients cope with psychological problems on prednisone? Dr. Lin had told me that a psychiatrist was now a part of the BMT team. Exactly what were they doing differently now for the long-term care of their patients? The Maynard bone marrow transplant website listed a "Cancer Survivorship" component of their support services, which appeared to address the long-term follow-up recommendations from the study. However, when I followed the link, I was routed to the page of general cancer support services offered to all cancer patients which included yoga and massage classes, nothing specifically related to the "specialized multidisciplinary management of both physician and psychiatrist" recommended by researchers.

I was recently contacted by the California-based activist group Consumer Watchdog, and I agreed to represent my District of San Luis Obispo County to advocate for better psychiatric monitoring by health professionals of patients on prescribed drugs that can cause mental disorders. There will be meetings. There will be speaking engagements. There will be visits to Sacramento where I and many others will tell our stories to our state representatives. The insurance companies and drug companies will try to block us. The California Medical Board will try to block us. But we will prevail because ultimately our stories are very simple to understand, and we speak for millions.

Bibliography

Boston Collaborative Drug Surveillance Program, The. 1972. "Acute Adverse Reactions to Prednisone in Relation to Dosage." *Clinical Pharmacology & Therapeutics* 13 (5part1): 694-698. doi:10.1002/cpt1972135part1694.

Cerullo, Michael. 2006. "Corticosteroid-Induced Mania: Prepare for the Unpredictable." *Current Psychiatry* 5 (6): 43-50. doi:10.1177/0091217415612735.

Fardet, Laurence, Irene Petersen, and Irwin Nazareth. 2012. "Suicidal Behavior and Severe Neuropsychiatric Disorders Following Glucocorticoid Therapy in Primary Care." *American Journal of Psychiatry* 169 (5): 491-497. doi:10.1176/appi.ajp.2011.11071009.

"Firearms: Shooting Yourself. Information on Suicide by Using a Gun." 2018. *Lostallhope.com*. http://lostallhope.com/suicide-methods/firearms.

"How to Recognize the Warning Signs of Suicide." 2018. *Wikihow*. https://www.wikihow.com/Recognize-the-Warning-Signs-of-Suicide.

Judd, Lewis L., Pamela J. Schettler, E. Sherwood Brown, Owen M. Wolkowitz, Esther M. Sternberg, Bruce G. Bender, and Karen Bulloch et al. 2014. "Adverse Consequences of Glucocorticoid Medication: Psychological, Cognitive, and Behavioral Effects." *American Journal of Psychiatry* 171 (10): 1048. doi:10.1176/appi.ajp.2014.13091264.

Sun, Can-Lan, Liton Francisco, K. Scott Baker, Daniel J. Weisdorf, Stephen J. Forman, and Smita Bhatia. 2011. "Adverse Psychological Outcomes in Long-Term Survivors of Hematopoietic Cell Transplantation: A Report from the Bone Marrow Transplant Survivor Study (BMTSS)." *Blood* 118 (17): 4723-4731. doi:10.1182/blood-2011-04-348730.

Warrington, Thomas P., and J. Michael Bostwick. 2006. "Psychiatric Adverse Effects of Corticosteroids." *Mayo Clinic Proceedings* 81 (10): 1361-1367. doi:10.4065/81.10.1361.

www.ingramcontent.com/pod-product-compliance
Lightning Source LLC
Chambersburg PA
CBHW030115100526
44591CB00009B/406